Far from Home

Far From HOME

Shattering the Myth of the Model Minority

MARY CHUNG HAYASHI

Founder of the National Asian Women's Health Organization

TAPESTRY PRESS
IRVING, TEXAS

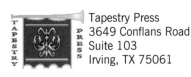 Tapestry Press
3649 Conflans Road
Suite 103
Irving, TX 75061

Printed in the USA
07 06 05 04 03 1 2 3 4 5

Library of Congress Cataloging-in-Publication Data

Hayashi, Mary Chung, 1967-
    Far from home : shattering the myth of the model minority / by
Mary Chung Hayashi.
        p. ; cm.
    Includes bibliographical references and index.
    ISBN 1-930819-32-3 (alk. paper)
    1. Asian Americans--Health and hygiene--Miscellanea. 2. Asian
Americans--Health and hygiene--Anecdotes. 3. Transcultural medical
care. 4. Health attitudes--Cross-cultural studies. 5. Health
behavior--Cross-cultural studies. 6. Asians--Health and
hygiene--Anecdotes. 7. Health promotion--Cross-cultural studies.
[DNLM: 1. Asian Americans--United States--Personal Narratives. 2.
Health Behavior--ethnology--United States--Personal Narratives. 3.
Attitude to Health--ethnology--United States--Personal Narratives. 4.
Health Education--United States--Personal Narratives. 5. Health
Promotion--United States--Personal Narratives. 6. Women's
Health--United States--Personal Narratives. WA 300 H413f 2003] I.
Title.
    RA448.5.A83H39 2003
    362.1'089'95073--dc22
                                        2003020548

Cover by David Sims
Book design and layout by
D. & F. Scott Publishing, Inc.
N. Richland Hills, Texas

To keeping hope alive, and to my family:

my sister Bo Yoon,
who never got to have an American name;
my younger sister Cindy
and her children Nick and John;
my brothers Phil and Peter and their families;
my parents;
and
the love of my life, my husband Dennis.

Contents

Introduction

Breaking the Silence

I remember a photograph that was taken of my sister and brother and me around 1972. We're on vacation somewhere in South Korea, holding hands and smiling for my father, who was taking the snapshot. I was five years old and was not called Mary then but Chung Mi Kyung. My older brother, Phil, was then Pil Ho. Our older sister, Bo Yoon, never had an American name. When I was twelve, she was cut out of the photograph.

Bo Yoon was my best friend. Growing up in the small town of Kwangju and later Seoul, I thought we were happy and close. But Bo Yoon was four years older than I was, and, at the time, I wasn't aware that she was having tremendous problems with depression. Depression—or really any health problem—was just not talked about in our family or our culture. Because Bo Yoon's struggle was a silent one, we were all completely shocked when on January 1, 1980 she took her own life.

That very day, all of her clothing and belongings were burned. Like the photograph, my parents and relatives tried to cut her memory from our family. There was never a funeral for

Bo Yoon, and our family still doesn't talk about her suicide or the mental illness that left her feeling so desperate.

Six months later, I was no longer Mi Kyung. I was Mary, a twelve-year-old Korean American girl who spoke no English. My father had moved us to Orange County, California. As a teenager experiencing culture shock, I began to feel the intense conflict between traditional Korean values and the freewheeling American culture of the early 1980s. It was a revelation. As I learned more about the American women's movement, I realized that I had the opportunity to reject certain cultural attitudes toward women and girls that had kept me from being independent.

I began to understand that my sister couldn't seek help because we were taught to keep our personal problems to ourselves. Clearly she had been struggling. The morning she hung herself in our room she showed me packages of sleeping pills she had taken. But I was too young to help her then, and, even if I had been older, I would have been held back by those around us who celebrated silence as strength.

For far too many years, Asian Americans from a wide variety of cultures have been considered the "model minority." Though we are all from distinct countries and regions with their own ethnic identities, since the 1960s, we have been statistically identified as Asian Americans. This label was in part of our own making since we do share similar culture, values, and challenges. As the model minority, we are considered successful and hardworking. We're the ones who are good at math, the Nobel Prize winning scientists. Our kids are honor-roll scholars and Westinghouse awards winners. We have close-knit families and communities. We eat healthy diets. We are smarter, more talented, better disciplined, better adjusted, play the violin really well, and, to many observers, are just plain healthier than other people of color as well as the white majority.

After high school, while working my way through college, I began to see that the myth of the model minority was pervasive and blinding. Few people outside the Asian American community realized how wrong it was. But I knew. I had lived behind the façade. I had kept the secret of my sister's suicide. And I saw a population at risk. I saw a disenfranchised community cut off from the help it needed by prejudice, language barriers, and its own cultural attitudes.

When it comes to health, we are all at risk. But we are not all at risk equally. So-called "mainstream Americans"—the majority, the white middle class—have big health advantages. Many years have been devoted to researching the threats to their health and what causes them. Government, health organizations, and the media target them with information and encouragement to modify risky behaviors and adopt a more healthful lifestyle. Research shows that they better understand the benefits of prevention, early detection, and researching all options for treatment than do minorities. A larger percentage of them have health insurance. They know that resources are available if they or someone in their family needs help. Even if they don't know the web site or telephone number for every need, more of them know how to find it.

All of this knowledge has reduced overall health risks for those who reside in the middle of that demographic bell curve. And that's what you would expect in America.

But with a population of 270 million, the number of people at the trailing ends of that curve—the people who face health risks without a safety net of knowledge, resources, and support—is in the tens of millions, and growing.

This book addresses eleven million of them—the Asian Americans. I am one of the roughly two-thirds of all Asian

Americans now living in this country that immigrated here. About half of those who are here feel that they don't speak English very well. They often feel isolated from the world around them, and so they cling to each other and to their traditional cultural values and attitudes.

Though the term is used to group us together, Asian Americans identify themselves as Asian Americans and Pacific Islanders as well as more than forty other ethnic subgroups. Now 4 percent of the US population, the Asian American population is expected to double within the next three decades. About 54 percent of Asian Americans live in the western United States, primarily in California and Hawaii, with 18 percent living in the Northeast, 17 percent in the South, and 11 percent in the Midwest.

While the majority of Asian Americans were born outside of the United States, many Chinese and Japanese Americans are fourth and fifth generation Americans. Since the mid-1960s, the population has grown rapidly with high influx from China, India, the Philippines, Korea, Vietnam, and Southeast Asia. Most Pacific Islanders are not immigrants, but are descendants of original inhabitants of territory taken over by the United States. This includes Hawaii, Tonga, Guam, American Samoa, the Northern Mariana Islands, the Marshall Islands, the Caroline Islands, and Palau.

Asian Americans and Pacific Islanders speak more than a hundred languages and dialects, with some ethnic groups experiencing more limited English proficiency than others: 61 percent of Hmong, 56 percent of Cambodian, 52 percent of Laotian, 44 percent of Vietnamese, 41 percent of Korean, and 40 percent of Chinese American households are isolated by their limited knowledge of the English language.

Socioeconomically, Asian American and Pacific Islanders run the gamut from the very rich to the very poor, from the most educated to the illiterate. In 2000, 44 percent of Asian American adults had a college or professional degree compared to 28 percent of white Americans. The majority of this group—58 percent—was South Asian Americans from India, Pakistan, Bangladesh, and Sri Lanka. In contrast, in 1990 only 12 percent of Hawaiians and 10 percent of other Pacific Islanders had completed college, and two of three Cambodian, Hmong, and Laotian American adults had not completed high school.

The average family income for Asian Americans and Pacific Islanders is higher than the national average, however we still experience a lower per capita income and higher rate of poverty than non-Hispanic white Americans. In 1990, about 14 percent of the whole AA/PI group was living in poverty, compared to 13.5 percent of all Americans, and 9 percent of non-Hispanic whites. Poverty rates for Asian Americans and Pacific Islanders ranged from a low of 6 percent for Filipino Americans to a high of 64 percent among Hmong Americans.

Among Asian American traditions is the silence that keeps problems, opinions, and complaints seething beneath the surface. I was born in Korea and learned from the moment I could talk that worries and problems were not to be discussed outside the family—and often not at all. Physical ailments are to be kept private. Mental disorders are shameful. There is no place for public discussion of a personal matter like health. Research is an intrusion. Advocating public policy is unthinkable.

In 1993, there was very little investigation into the health crisis facing Asian Americans, largely because no one thought there was anything to investigate. I knew differently.

This memoir not only shares my journey from South Korea to America but also from a helpless bystander to an advocate for Asian American health issues, first as founder of the National Asian Women's Health Organization (NAWHO) in 1993, and later as the national campaign director for the American Public Health Organization's "Campaign to Eliminate Health Disparities." Through my personal experience, anecdotes from the women's health community, and important NAWHO public education and research programs, this book dispels the myth of the model minority that puts those eleven million Asian Americans at risk.

While there are certainly gaps in the profile of the Asian American community, we have made great strides in the past decade to throw back the cloak of silence that keeps the community at risk. We have established enough facts to demonstrate how serious and widespread the problems are. Just consider a few of them:

- In Asia, women have some of the lowest incidence rates in the world for breast and cervical cancers. But when they migrate to the United States, the risk for these cancers increases six fold.
- Less than half of Asian women over the age of fifty have had a clinical breast examination and mammogram within the past two years—the lowest screening rate among all women.
- Sixty-five percent of Asian American women display low bone mineral density, the highest rate of all racial groups. More than one-fifth of Asian American women has osteoporosis.
- Asian American women over the age of sixty-five have the highest female suicide mortality rate, and adolescent girls have the highest rate of depressive symptoms of all racial and ethnic gender groups.
- The Asian American population is disproportionately affected by diabetes, which is the fifth leading cause of

death for Asian Americans between the ages of forty-five and sixty-four.

+ Asian American children are at twenty times the risk for infection from hepatitis B as other American children.

+ One in five Vietnamese and Korean Americans don't know that smoking causes heart and lung diseases and cancer.

+ Overall, Asian American men have the second-highest smoking rate of all male racial groups. One-third of Asian American women are exposed to secondhand smoke in the home or workplace everyday. Nearly one-quarter of Asian American high school-aged boys and 14 percent of the high school-aged girls smoke.

+ Eighty percent of Asian American men feel they are not at risk for HIV or, for that matter, any sexually transmitted diseases (STDs). Sixty percent have never been tested for HIV. Almost half do not always protect themselves against STDs and unplanned pregnancies.

+ Lack of health insurance keeps many Asian Americans from seeking preventive health care, and uninsured rates vary widely across Asian American populations. According to a 2001 study by The Commonwealth Fund, one in five Asian American adults between the ages of eighteen and sixty-four was uninsured or had been uninsured at some point in the past year, with especially high rates for Korean and Vietnamese Americans.

So much for the model minority.

Like other people from around the world, Asians come to America to find a new and better life. What they don't bargain for is the jarring culture shock they encounter and its destructive effects on their health. As a result, the fastest-growing segment of the US population suffers some of this country's worst health problems.

Perhaps the most important work of the last decade has been the process of empowering Asian American women and teaching them to take the risk of voicing their opinions. In 1998, 1999, and 2000, NAWHO became the first organization to provide an opportunity for young Asian American women and men to become leaders in health advocacy and public policy. Each year, the NAWHO National Leadership Network brought a hundred emerging Asian American health advocates to Washington, DC, to meet with members of Congress and others who shape public policy.

One woman at a time, one community at a time, we are building a new culture that emphasizes self-esteem and discards the tradition of silent suffering that works against health and well being. "Far From Home" is a wakeup call for Asian Americans. The risks have been identified. Now is the time for health care and social services professionals and, perhaps most importantly, Asian American women to educate their communities about disease prevention and healthy lifestyles. It's also the time for Asian Americans to reject stereotypically "Asian" nonassertiveness ("the nail that sticks up gets pounded down") and make their voices heard. Only then will policymakers work to provide leadership and funding for the research and assistance programs needed to reverse the deteriorating health of Americans of Asian descent.

More recently, as founder of the Iris Alliance Fund, I have focused my work on promoting the mental health of all children and families. From my experience in losing my sister, I have learned that my family is far from alone in suffering from the silence and stigma surrounding suicide. Today I can say, "My sister had a mental illness." And I hope by speaking out that I can help other families break the silence that keeps them from seeking professional help. I share my story—and my sister's story—to raise public awareness about the risks of mental illness. Our nation loses thirty thousand lives to suicide each year, and one in thirteen high school kids attempt suicide. The Iris Fund is working to break down misperceptions and eliminate stigma and discrimination surrounding this issue, which is a major public health issue in this country.

In 1993, when I founded NAWHO, few members of the Asian American establishment discouraged me from speaking out about the needs of our community. At first I questioned my decision. Should I keep quiet and obey these leaders, or should I move forward with what I knew to be important work? When my older sister told me about her depression, I had followed the old ways and kept quiet. But when I founded NAWHO, I knew that it was time for me to take my own road, to start the organization and work for positive change.

Throughout my life, I feel that I am continuously brought back to those core lessons of my early childhood training and that choice of whether or not to break the silence. Over the past ten years, as NAWHO has grown to include four thousand members and supporters in twenty-five states and the District of Columbia, many voices have joined together to send a strong message: In our increasingly diverse society, we must work together to reduce health disparities and build a healthy future for all Americans.

From 1998 through 2003, NAWHO has funded more than $1.1 million in grants to local organizations all over the country to launch Asian American women's health projects, empowering communities to reach their own constituencies.

By writing this book, I am again making the choice to use my voice. By doing so, I hope to inspire other women to write their own destinies and to see that we do not have to be controlled by our backgrounds, ethnicities, or family histories.

I Was Mi Kyung

When I close my eyes and think of Kwangju, the town in South Korea where I was born, I can feel the bite of the wind on my face and the warmth of my older sister's hand as we ice skated on the Geukrak River. Skating was one of our favorite pastimes, and, though there were safer places to skate, our first choice was always the river. On clear days it attracted children and adults alike with the promise of hours of exhilarating fun.

Kwangju is beautiful. Surrounded by high mountains, it lies in a natural river basin that has provided fertile land for farmers for many centuries. Today it's a thriving metropolitan area, the capital of the Chollanam-Do province. Kwangju calls itself the "City of Hope and Light," and it certainly fulfilled the hopes and dreams of my father.

We didn't have a lot of money when we lived in Kwangju. My father, Chung Yeon Sang had lost his own father in the Korean War and grew up in a nearby farming community with his mother. There he learned early on to be resourceful to support his family. He and my mother met in Kwangju in 1961. He was teaching Chinese, she was a student, and they fell in love. At the time, arranged marriages were the norm in Korea, and my mother's family, which owned land and had significant means, would never have chosen my father for their daughter. After all, she was a promising young tennis star, and, from their perspective, he was from a poor family with little to offer.

But my parents were strong headed. So, despite all objections and the fact that my mother's family refused to attend the wedding, they married when my mom was only twenty and my dad was twenty-nine. When my parents would tell us this story of their wedding, they did so with intense pride in their independence and opposition to authority. This show of free spirit belies the stereotype of the "passive" Asian but is actually considered part of the Kwangju mindset. I've often wondered if this atypical ancestral characteristic contributed to my own fierce independence.

For centuries the Kwangju people have fought for a place of recognition and importance. Once a region that was home only to farmers and pro-democracy activists, even in the last century, Kwangju has had to take a back seat to Seoul, which is considered the economic and spiritual heart of South Korea. Two incidents of the twentieth century illustrate the modern version of this willful mindset. First in 1929, when Japan occupied Korea, Kwangju students mounted vocal demonstrations against discrimination and colonial rule. Again in 1980, the citizens of Kwangju rose up against General Chun Doo Hwan's assumption of power. They advocated a stronger people's democracy.[1]

Charged with this spirit of the city, my father transformed himself into a young entrepreneur in the 1960s full of ideas for making money in South Korea's budding democratic economy. Though few people had enough money to buy cars, and even fewer cars were available for purchase in South Korea at the time, he could see that the future would be far different. So my father opened the first gas station in Kwangju. That was the beginning of his long and successful career as a business-man and president of several of his own companies.

While my father was starting out in business, eight of us—my parents, my siblings and I, and my father's mother—lived in a three-bedroom rental house. Two of the bedrooms were connected, making one large room with a par-tial wall separating the space. Here my grandmother and the five children—my sister, Bo Yoon, the eldest, my older brother, Pil Ho, my younger sister and brother, Il Yung and Pil Sun, and I—all slept together. The kitchen was connected to the bedroom, and the stove provided some heat in the win-ter. I also remember that we bought charcoals and put them underneath the floor to warm the room. Sometimes we all got sick from the fumes of this antiquated heating method or the occasional gas leak, and my grandmother would make us some clear *kim-chee* broth as a cure-all.

As was the custom, my siblings and I were born in that home with the help of a midwife. Only my older brother was born in a hospital because he arrived prematurely. While we didn't have a close relationship with my mother's side of the family, we always seemed to have one relative or another from my father's side of the family living with us—not only my grandmother, but also for many years my cousin Soon Oak, whose parents couldn't afford to take care of her. This wasn't unusual in our community, because many families struggled to keep food on the table.

When I was seven years old, and we were still living in Kwangju, I had to go to the doctor every day for a year. I had chronic sinus problems, so, every day after school I took the bus to the doctor's office. By American standards, this might seem ambitious for a seven-year-old, but though Kwangju is a city of over 1.3 million people today, in the early 1970s, it was still a small town. Everyone knew me, and I knew them. There was only one doctor's office in the whole city, and it was impossible to get lost.

There was a nurse in the office that always greeted me enthusiastically and seemed to like me a lot. She made a point to tell my parents that I was the best little girl and didn't cry when I got my shots every day. Strangely, though, I don't ever remember saying more than one or two words to her and don't even remember her name. I would greet her with a timid hello, and every day she would ask me if I wanted something to eat. I would tell her simply, "No," and this was the extent of our conversations. Still she would tell my parents that I was brave and that I was a "good girl." In my family, and truly throughout the Asian culture, this is the ultimate compliment.

My father and my grandmother taught me early on that one of the most important virtues was to be a "good girl." In Korea, as it is in so many Asian cultures, more than anything else, being a good girl meant keeping my mouth shut and my thoughts and opinions to myself. Any kind of direct communication—even direct eye contact—was discouraged. Avoiding conflict altogether was pervasive in the culture and was expected of both girls and boys.

Growing up in this way, my sisters and I were taught that we had to be good girls because we were always representing the family. There was no "I," only "we" and "the family." We had to be good girls or we would shame our parents. As a result, we carried around a heavy burden to be perfect that I believe is at the root of some of the significant health risks Asian American women face today.

As I grew up, I began to notice that this emphasis on "family" overshadowed individual rights and achievements. Men were not men until they got married. Then they were defined by their jobs. My father, for instance was always called "Mr. President" not Mr. Chung. Women were not respected until they became mothers, and even then they did not have their own identity but would be called "Mother of Mi Kyung." Truly being a mother was the ultimate goal for girls since little opportunity existed for careers or an individual place of respect in society outside of the family.

While Asian parents do tend to be strong advocates for education, and this was certainly true for my parents, this desire extended exclusively to my brothers, who were encouraged to pursue a higher education to help them in business. My sisters and I, however, were only encouraged to be "good girls" and to go to school long enough to marry someone wealthy before we were twenty-one and over the hill.

Passiveness was a natural byproduct of being a good girl. Bo Yoon and I were not troublemakers. We respected our elders, never talked back, and, for the most part, obeyed the rules. When we did disobey, we made sure we didn't get caught. Skating on the river, for instance, was all the more thrilling to us because we were supposed to skate at the skating rinks, which were certainly safer. As young girls living within these parameters, I thought we were happy. Korea is a remarkably homogenous culture—there was no one showing us that there was another way to live. It was a simple life.

But when put in the context of the American culture, this behavior was—and still is—widely promoted among not only Asian girls but girls from a number of cultural backgrounds. In her groundbreaking book *Odd Girl Out*, Rachel Simmons points out that even the American culture "refuses girls access to open conflict."

"Silence is deeply woven into the fabric of the female experience," she writes.[2]

By the time we moved to Seoul in 1978, when I was eleven years old, the culture of silence was firmly ingrained in both Bo Yoon and me. We were prosperous, living in a large house my father had designed himself. My mother was an anomaly, by this time a talented professional tennis player, gone much of the time to play in tournaments.

Everything in Seoul was about appearances.

Our house in Seoul was beautiful with large windows and marble walls. We had our own garage, which was rare and envied. And we always had dogs, which was another visible sign of prosperity. Our neighborhood had no backyards—everything was in front and on display. From the outside, all looked happy and prosperous, but inside there were many problems.

As far back as I can remember, my parents were unhappy in their relationship. One day when I was about five and we were still living in Kwangju, I went into my mother's room to play with the makeup and cold cream on her dressing table. I thought she was sleeping, but she turned to me and asked me if she and my father split up whether I would go with her or stay with my dad.

Sometimes I would see them together, and they would be acting so happy. But those happy times dwindled the more my mother played tennis. She was only a professional for one season.

One thing that I loved about our big new house in Seoul was that I still shared a room with my older sister. Even though she was four years older than I was, we were close. I thought that everything about her was wonderful—she was tall and was popular. She was a cheerleader. She was smart, but she had to study hard because in Korea at that time it was extremely difficult for girls to get into the university. My parents always stressed to us the importance of getting into a university so that we would increase our chances of meeting and marrying an educated man.

When we were little, every year on New Year's Day, all of us would dress up in our best clothes and go to our relatives' houses and do a formal bow. Then they would give us money. But in 1979 and 1980, we no longer did this because our relatives were three hundred miles away in Kwangju. So on January 1, 1980, I had the day to myself without family plans. I was getting ready to go to a friend's house when Bo Yoon told me she wanted to tell me something, but only if I promised not to share it with anyone. Of course I agreed to keep her secret.

"Look in the garbage can," she told me.

There in the bottom were all of these over-the-counter sleeping pill wrappers.

"What did you do?" I asked. "What's going on?"

"I can't take it any more," she said. "Last night was too hard for me. I needed something."

We were all afraid of my father, who we thought was perfect and who we knew expected perfection from us. Bo Yoon made me promise that I would not tell our father. Of course I promised her that I wouldn't tell. And then I went on to my friend's house as planned.

As cold as Kwangju could be in the winter, Seoul was far colder, and that day was gray, windy and raining. As I left the house, my grandmother and I quarreled because it was a holiday, and, even though we weren't observing the New Year's tradition, she thought that I should be with the family. But I left anyway.

At about 1:00 PM, the phone rang at my friend's house. It was Soon Oak, my cousin, who still lived with us in Seoul. As soon as the phone rang, I knew it was about my sister, even though all that Soon Oak said was that my dad wanted me to come home immediately. I could feel that something terrible had happened.

It was still raining when I got on the bus, and I just stared out the window in a daze thinking about what my sister had told me that morning. Before I knew it, I had missed the bus stop for our house. I had to get off the bus and walk quite a long way home. When I got there, I learned that my older brother, Pil Ho, had found Bo Yoon hanging in our room. I wanted to see her, but her body and all of her belongings had already been removed from the house.

The next day, my brothers and sister and I were sent away to Kwangju to our Auntie's. There was no funeral for my sister, and neither of my parents ever talked to us about the suicide. We never celebrated Christmas or New Year's again as a family.

Now twenty-three years later, I think that my sister was trying to tell me that life was too hard for her at seventeen, that she was under too much pressure, and that she had nowhere to turn for help but to over-the-counter sleeping pills. Now I know that our culture didn't leave room for good girls to feel so desperate, or at least to express that desperation. Asking for help would only bring shame upon the family. But Bo Yoon's cryptic words—that life was too hard for her—meant little to me at twelve.

My parents separated shortly after my sister's suicide, and our family never seemed whole again. I don't even have a picture of Bo Yoon, because all of the photographs of her were burned along with her clothes. But I do have the picture that was taken of us on summer vacation. My brother and I are still smiling at the camera and holding hands. And even though someone cut Bo Yoon out of the picture, I know that she was there, holding my hand and smiling, too.

Years after my sister died, I was looking at a cute picture of my younger sister. It was taken on our last family vacation in Korea. We were all out on a boat. It was after my older sister had died. My older brother glanced at the picture in my hand and remarked that it was taken where he and my parents had scattered my older sister's ashes.

"How strange," I thought. Why would my parents take us back there on a vacation of all places? Had they really erased her so thoroughly from their memory, or were they somehow trying to include her? Of course I wouldn't know because the subject has always been entirely taboo. It took me two decades to talk about it and to break the silence that I had learned was so virtuous, that was the hallmark of the good girl.

When my sister died, I was a good girl. I was still Mi Kyung. But only a few short months after her death, a whole new life began for me in America as Mary.

CHAPTER TWO

Journey to America

When we moved to America in 1980, I had just turned thirteen. We settled in Orange County in a quintessential American neighborhood. The Brady Bunch could have lived on our street it was so typically upper middle class. These nice suburban houses with neat yards were home to girls that looked just like 1980s versions of Marsha and Jan.

I didn't speak a word of English on my first day at Hewes Junior High School and I walked into a classroom where blonde California girls surrounded me. There were no African Americans in our school, and I was one of only five Asians.

I didn't understand a thing on that first day of seventh grade. Before we came to the United States, I had only begun to learn the English alphabet in school. At the time, there were some English as Second Language (ESL) programs in the US public school system. Later I learned that my Korean friends in Los Angeles had been offered ESL classes, but since my school was so homogenous, there hadn't been a need in the past. So, I perfected invisibility. I guess you could say that the Korean culture was good training for this because I was used to living in silence.

I realized early on that all I had to do to get by was just sit quietly and listen. While I was lost in most subjects, math was easy for me because the math classes I had taken in Korea put me a couple of years ahead of the US curriculum. The kids in the school were really nice to me—after all, I was a novelty. We did have one nasty neighbor who used to tell us to "go home." I had a black German Shepherd that went everywhere with me, and this neighbor would turn the hose on us on a regular basis. Welcome to America!

The second semester of that year, I had a math teacher who made me really uncomfortable because she regularly made students explain problems in front of the whole class. Every day I sat there petrified that she would pick me and I wouldn't know what to say. I did my best to avoid eye contact, but one day she called on me.

Though I certainly knew how to do the problem and knew the correct answer, I couldn't even begin to talk about it to the class. I just broke down and started crying. The teacher sent me to the office, and, thankfully, they called in a Korean boy to translate for me. I poured my heart out to him and told him how frustrated I was because I was afraid that my teachers might think I wasn't very smart. My biggest fear at the time was that my math teacher might think that I wasn't obeying her rules. The fact that I couldn't follow her order to explain the math problem was the most upsetting for me.

"I'm not stupid," I told him. "I just can't speak English!"

It's unbelievable to me now that I could go almost six months in a school and have only a few people—several teachers and the student who had the locker below mine—notice that I couldn't speak the language. Although you might think my father should have paved the way and talked to the school about getting me some extra help, he never would have thought about doing such a thing because he would have viewed that as a sign of weakness. My dad was intensely proud of being Korean. Though he chose American names for all of us when we moved—I became Mary; my older brother Pil Ho became Phil; my younger brother Pil Sun became Peter; and my little sister Il Yung became Cindy—my dad always used his traditional three-part Korean name, Chung Yeon Sang. And though he moved us to America, he still preferred that we keep the Korean customs and seek out other Koreans as friends.

I was worried that my dad would find out that I had been crying at school and sent to the office. And so I hid the math class incident from him. When the school got me a tutor to help with my English, I downplayed it. But the tutor helped a lot, and I started to get enthused about my studies. In the eighth grade, I made the honor roll both semesters. I was now living the myth of the model minority.

It was strange to me that the school was so eager—once they found out—to provide me with help. In Korea, the private junior high and high school we went to were extremely strict. We wore black skirts and bright, clean white collars. Each day, when we walked through the doors of the school, teachers were waiting to make sure our hair was not longer than two centimeters below our ears. We all had to have the same strait, blunt haircut, and, if you happened to have naturally curly hair, you had to straiten it every day or you would get slapped. If you dared to ever cry in class or talk back to a teacher, you faced physical discipline.

Since my parents had separated not long after my sister's suicide, my mother didn't initially come to America with us. When my parents divorced—and then later briefly got back together—I never told anyone. Even though divorce was more typical in my American community, the Korean belief system was still ruling my thoughts. My mother had taken us to

Catholic Church in Korea. In that community, divorce was still a huge stigma and something that was looked down upon. It was fine to stay married and live your entire life miserable together, because being divorced was as bad as having cancer—it was abhorred.

In America, I was the oldest daughter in a household without a mother, so I was the one expected to cook and clean and do the laundry for the family. Our house was quite large with four bedrooms, and, to this day, I hate doing housework because I had so much of it forced upon me for so many years. I remember that it impressed people when they found out that I had learned to make *kim-chee*, a Korean spicy hot fermented pickle seasoned with garlic, chilies, onion, ginger, and other spices. I also learned to make my brothers and sister macaroni and cheese! One of my favorite chores was going to the supermarket. We had a Ralph's near our house, and, compared to doing the grocery shopping in Korea—which still involved stops at several different kinds of stores, the convenience and choices of product at Ralph's impressed me.

The positive tradeoff to my responsibilities was that, other than my dad, I was the boss of the household. None of my siblings bucked me because they knew that I was the one taking care of them. To this day, I still have that role in the family to some extent and, if anything bad happens to any of them, I feel at least partly responsible.

I certainly don't think that my father ever believed he was mistreating me by heaping on the responsibility. I think he was truly proud of me. When I was fourteen, he bought me a grand piano because he wanted me to continue playing. In Korea, my older sister and I, my older brother, and my mother had all taken lessons.

The major break from the workload, though, was going to church on Sundays, where I played the piano during services.

For the first few years that I was in America, the Orange County Korean Baptist Church was my entire social life. My family was pretty isolated in Orange County, and the Korean church helped us find friends and support. We went to church on Sundays and to Bible study meetings on Wednesday evenings. On Saturdays, I looked for every opportunity to be at church for an organized activity or even just to baby-sit small children while their mothers were in church meetings.

The church was a total support system for my family. We learned how to study for driver's license exams, what kind of credit cards would be most useful, and where all the good Korean restaurants were in Orange County. Sometime the church people would take us to the Black Angus steak house. Back in Korea, we were always told that meat was precious and rare, so being able to eat large steaks was a real treat.

Church was where I met my first close girlfriend, Sunny, who was a huge influence in my life. Sunny invited me to take oil painting classes with her, which I loved then and still enjoy. She also invited me to partake of that great American teenage pastime—the mall. And we often went camping together with other kids from church.

Sunny was four years older than I was—the same age as my older sister. She had her own car, so I was able to go just about anywhere with her. When Sunny moved to the San Francisco Bay Area to attend college, I was very sad. But we stayed in touch, and, eventually, I decided to move up to the Bay Area as well.

When I first moved to America, I remember that I was so happy every time I saw Connie Chung on television. Here was this woman who was beautiful and articulate and successful in her profession on national television. I remember telling my dad that I wanted to be just like her. She was the one Asian person that I connected with, and I thought she was amazing.

Her success began to open my own eyes to the opportunities that were available to me.

By the time I was a freshman at Foothills High School, I could clearly see that the rules at my house were far different from most. We all had to be home before dark, and, in the wintertime when the sun set early, that was a problem. Neither my little sister nor I was allowed to have a boyfriend. Makeup was definitely not allowed. And so I began to live a double life—that of the good girl at home, the little mother taking care of her family, as well as the life of an independent teenage girl trying to find a place for herself.

I would go to school early every day so that I could put on my makeup—complete with fake eyelashes to make my eyes look more Anglo. I tried to dye my hair blonde, which turned it a bizarre shade of red. I started smoking cigarettes when I was sixteen; I thought this made me look more American.

Using makeup, changing my hair color, smoking—these were the things that I thought would make me fit in with the white kids in my school. But none of these things made me feel good about myself.

I felt like my dad didn't understand who I was or anything about the American culture. He fought hard against assimilation. He was frustrated with the whole American system. In Korea, daughters would live with their parents until they married. But in the United States, my father witnessed his friends' daughters living in college dorms or with their boyfriends. He didn't understand how parents could let their kids do this sort of thing.

My father also was increasingly concerned with trying to keep Korean customs alive in our family. I also think he was frustrated because he had lost a certain amount of status in America. In Korea, he was "Mr. President," but in America, he was still looking for his next business opportunity. Also, he had to rely on me to translate for him, which made him extremely uncomfortable. By this time, my mother had moved back in with us again, and the two of them decided that America was ruining their children.

So one day, my dad announced that we were going back home to Seoul. And just like that—all of my siblings packed up to leave. I wasn't about to go. I wanted to live my own life, to stay and take my chances. While my father was perfectly willing to pay for my brothers to attend college, I had been paying my own tuition to California State University Long Beach. This alone made me feel independent enough to tell my father that I wanted to stay in America. I think that in part because we hadn't sold our house yet, he agreed to let me stay. The only stipulation was that I would have to take care of the house and keep it in perfect order for the real estate agent to show.

In just a few short months, college began to open my eyes. I was reading a lot of feminist literature—Virginia Wolf, Sylvia Plath and others—and I was learning firsthand about the many opportunities for women in America that were impossibilities in Korea. I had become a citizen when I was eighteen, so I could vote, could work and support myself, go to college, and live on my own.

But my parents didn't quit trying to get me back into the fold. The first time I visited them after they had moved back, one of our relatives introduced me to a man in Korea that she and my father had chosen for me to marry. I went along with it for about six months. Park Han Chal was four years older than I was. He was from a wealthy family and didn't have to work. The only thing he did was go to the stock market each morning. After that he was free to do what he wanted. While I was visiting, we would spend time together in the afternoon. He wasn't a typical Korean since he spoke English pretty well and traveled a lot, so, I was open to it in the beginning. My mother went to see a fortuneteller and was told by her that Han and I were a good match. My family was thrilled.

Han liked to talk about his "American Dream" because he wanted to live in America. We were really just friends, but he did finally make it clear that he wanted to marry me. Reluctantly I agreed to meet his parents. My dad and I went with him and his parents to a traditional Korean restaurant in Seoul where you sit on the floor with your shoes off and are served many little dishes of every kind of meat and fish and vegetable. So, there we sat, when the future mother-in-law asked me a question.

"In America, I hear that women drive cars. Is this true? Do you drive?" she asked.

I was about to answer in Korean, and this man I'm supposed to marry makes it clear that I'm not supposed to answer. I'd forgotten all about being a good girl! I'd lost touch with the odd dance that Korean women do where they aren't supposed to talk even if a question is directly asked of them! I had entirely forgotten that in this situation, the man was supposed to answer for the woman. And that's exactly what Han did.

After that night I knew that I couldn't go back and live the life of Mi Kyung. I was Mary now, and it was time for me to move forward.

CHAPTER THREE

On My Own

I'm sure many other women have had their own Helen Reddy "I am woman" moments. There comes a time when we just have to roar, when we're down there on the floor and decide that "no one's ever gonna keep me down again."

My moment probably came while I was cleaning my family's house in Orange County.

It's not the work itself that pushed me over the edge, but the fact that even when my family was on the other side of the Pacific Ocean, I found myself in their control. They were gone; I was ostensibly living on my own in the "Land of the Free." Yet I was still taking care of them. And I was doing it while working another full-time job to put myself through college. While my brothers were supported in their pursuit of higher education and meaningful professional work, my sister and I were advised to get married and have families of our own.

All of my friends from high school were going to college—even the ones who didn't get good grades. Yet, my father had never encouraged me to even apply. I actually did so only as an afterthought, just to follow the crowd. I ended up at California State University Long Beach (CSULB) because by the time I decided to go to college, that was the only school whose deadline I hadn't missed.

Even though I was continuing my education, I was really just going through the motions with little conscious direction. I had numerous jobs, from working at a restaurant as a hostess to doing secretarial work at a computer company.

Meanwhile, at CSULB, I signed up for a women's studies class. At the top of our reading list was Charlotte Bronte's *Jane Eyre*. When I finished reading about this woman who pursued her own dreams despite intense suffering, I truly felt like a weight had been lifted from my own shoulders. I felt like I was free to do anything. As I went on to learn about many of the leaders of the American feminist movement, perhaps for the first time in my life, I was truly excited about my own future.

In Korea, women weren't expected to get jobs. The be all and end all was meeting the right man and having his children. But as a young woman living on my own in America, I opened my eyes to see that there were many other possibilities. Suddenly I was energized by the realization that I could set my own goals and work toward them—even if I didn't have the full support of my family. I was ready to head out in a new direction. And since my friend Sunny had moved to the Bay Area, north seemed like a good direction at the time.

My first apartment was in Oakland. I loved that little studio apartment and was so happy that everything in it—my black couch and my futon—was my own. I still wanted to get a degree, so I enrolled in night classes at the University of San Francisco. I also started looking for a job.

My first job was as a bookkeeper with an Asian American civil rights organization. The Bay Area was a great place for emerging young activists to be, and I was motivated by the exciting work going on around me. There were many non-profits in the area with roots at the University of California Berkeley campus nearby. All of them were looking for volunteers, and I was willing.

For the first time I began to see myself as an "Asian American" and identify with the Asian American community. I poured my energy into learning more about the community, its history, and the social issues that were effecting it.

Up to this point I had not known a lot about the many ethnic groups that make up the Asian American community. At work and in the many volunteer jobs I began to take in my spare time, I met Asian Americans from different backgrounds and was inspired by their experiences. Working successfully within the Asian American community requires building coalitions and understanding the nuances of these distinct cultures. I began to appreciate the various contributions of Asian Americans and the fact that although we all come from different places, in America, we have to work together.

The stories of injustice driving the Asian American political movement were plentiful. I learned about the internment of Japanese Americans during World War II, about the plight of Chinese Americans and their role in building the railroads, and about Vietnamese fishermen and their mistreatment by the US Coast Guard.

The early 1990s were also a period of growth for the women's movement. I volunteered for the San Francisco chapter of the National Organization for Women, for various labor and reproductive rights organizations, as well as for Korean American women's projects and area battered women's shelters.

Even though I was naïve about the various causes and had limited skills, these groups welcomed my contributions and made me feel accepted and appreciated. I did anything and everything. I helped with bookkeeping for events, stuffed envelopes, sold fundraising tickets for dinners, and even did telemarketing to raise money and awareness.

I was so ready to work, to learn, and to change—not only myself but also the community around me. For the first time in my life, I was able to help others and myself. I watched women band together to discuss choice and women's health. They were speaking out for change, and their voices were making a difference. Together they were changing public policy and medical practice.

It was an exciting time for women's health; many organizations were forming to address women's health issues. But I was watching this happen everywhere except in my own Asian American community. African Americans, Latina women and Caucasian women were driving the movement, but Asian American women were visibly absent from the important social change that was happening at the time.

Women's movement leaders in the Bay Area as well as the leaders of national organizations for African American and Latina women also saw the void and began to encourage me to work on women's issues within the Asian American community. True, there was no national or statewide organization to speak for Asian American women, but who was I to start such an organization?

I had little money and truly lived month to month. I was still years away from getting a college degree. I was lonely and didn't have support from my family. Thankfully, my sister Cindy had moved back to Orange County in 1991, so I did have her encouragement—even though it came over the phone lines. Our phone bills from that time were enormous because we talked every day. (We still do!)

So in 1993, at age twenty-six, after working in the Asian American community for three years, I decided I would no longer be a silent bystander. Armed solely with inspiration from what was going on around me, I decided it was time to find my voice and to use it to create a national organization for Asian American women.

CHAPTER FOUR

Finding a Voice

Sometimes I think it's inaccurate for me to be called the "founder" of the National Asian Women's Health Organization (NAWHO), because, in many ways, I think the organization—or at least the need for it—found me.

I never consciously set out to be a leader of a movement, but I had learned that there was a need in the Asian American women's community for better awareness of and access to health care. So, I started talking about it and asking questions. Of course, no one came to my apartment to tell me, "This is how you build a movement." But I did have many role models for inspiration and guidance.

The early 1990s were an exciting time for women's health. In 1983, The United States Task Force on Women's Health was convened and began to evaluate the role of the US Department of Health and Human Services in women's health. Women's health had largely been uncharted territory until that time. Scientific knowledge about the prevention and treatment of diseases common in or unique to women was insufficient since research dollars and clinical trials had been largely focused on men. Among the task force's recommendations was to increase women's participation in research studies and clinical trials.

In response, in 1987, the National Institutes of Health (NIH) developed a new policy to include women in clinical trials and in 1990 established the Office of Research on Women's Health (ORWH) to identify gaps in knowledge and increase research. In 1991, the ORWH launched the Women's Health Initiative (WHI), which, for the first time, sought to address the most common causes of death, disability and impaired quality of life in postmenopausal women. The fifteen-year multi-million dollar effort became one of the largest US prevention studies of its kind. The overall goal of WHI was to reduce coronary heart disease, breast and colorectal cancer, and fractures due to osteoporosis by identifying risk factors and prevention strategies. While its goals were specific, the initiative attracted attention to women's health by other federal agencies as well as private organizations.

The WHI joined a collective voice advocating women's health issues that had been gaining strength for some years. In 1983, for instance, health activist Byllye Avery founded the National Black Women's Health Project (NBWHP) to improve the health status of African American women and promote their empowerment as educated health care consumers. In 1990, the organization reached an important milestone when it opened a Public Education and Policy office in Washington, DC. Byllye eventually became one of the original members of the NAWHO Board of Directors. And Julia Scott, NBWHP's director of public policy and later its president, and Cynthia Newbille, NBWHP's president at the time, really helped me on a day-to-day basis.

About the same time, the National Latina Health Organization was formed to raise consciousness about Latina health and health problems and encourage Latina women to take greater control of their health practices and lifestyles. This organization's executive director, Luz Alvarez-Martinez, was also generous with advice and support. She even let me use her offices in Oakland for a month as I was getting NAWHO started.

Dian Harrison, who has served in leadership positions with the United Way and the Urban League and is now president and CEO of Planned Parenthood of Golden Gate, was also a knowledgeable resource for NAWHO. Dian still helps me and has always inspired me to take action and not wait for others to solve problems.

So, following the example of these women of color, I began to explore starting an organization that would raise awareness of the health crisis among Asian Americans and empower Asian American women to organize, educate themselves, and pursue their own solutions to the health and social problems they face.

I knew that Asian Americans were not the first racial or ethnic group that found itself outside the health care system. African Americans and Hispanics had a similar history. With these ethnic groups, I had seen the government and health care professionals respond—albeit slowly and with much prodding from organizations like the National Black Women's Health Project and the National Latina Health Organization—with programs aimed at educating these populations and giving them better access to appropriate care.

But the situation that Asian Americans faced was more complex. The Asian American community was one of the fastest growing racial or ethnic segments of the US population. To non-Asians, they were considered a monolithic racial and ethnic group respected for their self-discipline, hard work, academic excellence, entrepreneurial spirit, deep family and religious values, and strong community ties. But in fact, Asian Americans were a complex, diverse community encompassing more than forty distinct cultures and dozens of different languages and dialects.

As I tried to grow a list of supporters, I found many community and health care leaders who just didn't understand the need for an Asian American health organization. Again, they were buying into the stereotype—Asians were healthy people who ate tofu—and would just scratch their heads in wonder when I came to talk to them. So I had to build a case for support with the research and anecdotal support that existed.

The initial needs assessment I conducted told me that the specific health needs of Asian Americans had been overlooked and underestimated in large part because of stereotypes perpetuated by the myth of the model minority. I knew that this stereotype simply was not true for the vast numbers of Asians in the United States, and that it masked the enduring barriers to health care that many Asian Americans encountered. The lack of understanding about the health needs of this community was being complicated by the fact that Asian American women living in the United States came from such a variety of ethnic backgrounds, and had varying levels of English proficiency, cultural integration, and economic status. For example, at that time, approximately 14 percent of Asian Americans lived in poverty, but when broken down by ethnic group, the rates ranged from 65 percent for Hmong living in poverty to less than 10 percent for Japanese Americans. Southeast Asians in general had the highest welfare dependency rates of any ethnic or racial group.[1]

I knew that we had to work both within the Asian American community and with the mainstream preventive health care community to overcome the disparities. Asian Americans were particularly absent when it came to seeking preventive health care. According to a study by The Commonwealth Fund Commission on Women's Health, Asian women were the least likely to obtain clinical preventive services.[2]

In general, all Asian Americans have low rates of health care utilization, and they will only seek services if there is a serious problem where they can no longer function normally in their day-to-day lives. Western concepts of preventive medical care simply do not exist in Asian cultures. Consequently, many diseases such as cancer were being diagnosed at later stages, and as research was beginning to reveal, Asian Americans were more likely to use invasive and emergency care—making up over 18 percent of total emergency room visits, compared to about 12 percent for Caucasian Americans. Asian American women in particular make their own health and well-being less of a priority, as most Asian cultural norms dictate that they put the lives of their family members first.

For instance, screenings for cervical cancer are considered extremely cost-effective because the disease can be treated relatively easily in its early stages. However, many women in the Asian American community were not utilizing these early detection methods. Vietnamese women had an extremely high incidence rate for cervical cancer of 43 cases per 100,000. This is more than twice the rate of Hispanic women, which is the second highest for all racial groups at 16.2 per 100,000.[3]

Beyond these physical health issues, statistics also showed that a number of complex issues—violence, high social expectations and pressures, poverty, cultural adjustments, lack of family support, and post-traumatic stress disorder related to refugee experiences—combined to create high mental health needs for Asian Americans. In 1994, the National Center for Health Statistics indicated that Asian American women over the age of sixty-five had the highest female suicide mortality rate among all ethnic and racial groups. Also, Asian Americans had the highest suicide mortality rate among all women between fifteen and twenty-four years of age.[4]

Still, I knew that few Asian Americans feel safe in accessing mental health care specialists, and, because many experience psychosomatic symptoms of stress and depression such as hypertension, ulcers, headaches, backaches, insomnia, and digestive problems, they will seek only primary health care, if any care at all.

I had my work cut out for me. Government and health care providers were largely unaware of the growing health crisis among Asian Americans in part due to the myth of the model minority but also because of the reticence of the Asian American community to communicate about health issues. Also, the tremendous diversity of languages and cultures within the Asian American community made it impossible to design one solution that fit all.

I knew that none of these problems could be solved without an organization to lead the way. So, I looked to those who had succeeded for help. The first time I talked to Julia Scott at the National Black Women's Health Project about whether I should start an organization for Asian American women, her response was an immediate "yes" followed by an enthusiastic "and I'm going to help you." Then she did something that I now know is rare in the nonprofit community—she began to share grant contacts to help me get NAWHO funded.

One of the first people Julia introduced me to was Jael Silliman at the Jessie Smith Noyes Foundation. Jael is an incredibly accomplished woman, scholar, and writer. A South Asian, who is also Jewish, she was born in Calcutta. Jael is one of the most positive people I know, as is evidenced by her initial reaction when I told her about what I was trying to do.

"Where have you been?" I remember her saying. "I've been looking for an Asian American women's organization to fund."

I really needed that kind of encouragement in those early days because even without a car payment or a mortgage, my financial cushion was thin. If NAWHO didn't get funded fast, I couldn't continue working to establish it. Jael went out of her way to make phone calls to other foundations on my behalf, and, after she left the foundation, she served as NAWHO Board chair for four years.

Another important grant contact that Julie and Cynthia shared with me was Shira Sapperstein at the Moriah Fund. By the time I went to see Shira in Washington, DC, I had been unemployed for some time and was completely broke. We had an early morning appointment that required me to fly in the night before, and paying for that hotel room was a real stretch for me. I stayed up late the night before the meeting preparing my spiel, going over my goals for the organization, the need for targeted research and education, and my long-term vision.

When I walked in to see Shira the next morning, before I could even get into my best material, she stopped me and said, "I get it. You need to exist. Now, how can I help?" Even though I still had to go back to San Francisco and write a proposal, Shira was on board.

The Moriah Fund's offices were in Maryland at the time, and I had a long cab ride ahead of me to get to the airport that day. Shira had dealt with fledgling nonprofit organizations long enough to know that the cab fare was going to be difficult for me. She offered to pay for the cab, but I wouldn't let her because I was too proud. Still, the gesture meant so much to me because it showed her level of support and her understanding of just how hard it was to get an organization like NAWHO off the ground. Then Shira went a step further. After she saw my proposal, she started calling other foundations on my behalf to help get NAWHO more funding. The doors started to open for NAWHO.

Initial grants of $25,000 from the Jesse Smith Noyes Foundation, $15,000 from the Moriah Fund and $10,000 from The Sister Fund ensured that NAWHO was on its way. I'm proud to say that all of these foundations became long-time supporters of NAWHO.

While I received encouragement and inspiration from many individuals and organizations, oddly enough, I faced opposition from within my own Asian American community. A few members of the Asian American establishment were questioning the need for an initiative dedicated to Asian women's health and were discouraging me from speaking out about the needs of Asian woman and families. They were even quietly talking to others to discourage them from supporting NAWHO.

It's rarely publicly acknowledged, but there is a definite hierarchy at work in the Asian American community where long-established community leaders are looked to as spokespeople. It was difficult for someone like me, relatively unknown and only twenty-six, to be taken seriously by the leadership and the community as a whole. Though initially I did question my decision to start NAWHO, I no longer wanted to be passive and silent. I wanted to have a voice and create an organization to help people.

We have left our countries and come to America, but sometimes it's hard to leave behind our culture. I did not want to be ruled by the old ways that taught me to be silent. I was determined to move forward with what I knew to be important work even if I had to do so without everyone's support.

For many Asian Americans, personal and family health is such an intensely private matter that they view professional health care largely as a last resort, sought only in the case of grave illness. They look to traditional Asian beliefs about diseases and disease prevention to be reliable, and live largely in denial of their health risks. They don't realize their risks or what health care opportunities are available. And even when they do, their cultural traditions keep them from getting the help they need.

I couldn't help but think back to the day when my older sister had told me about her depression. I had followed the old ways and kept quiet then. This time, I would not choose to be passive. In many ways, I founded NAWHO for those women who were discouraging me as well as for all of the Asian American women who could not let go of a culture that was keeping them silent.

I admired congresswoman Patsy Mink for many reasons. In 1965, she became the first Asian American woman to be elected to the US Congress and for four decades was a vocal advocate for women's rights and for Asian Americans. As a member of the Education and Workforce and Budget and Steering Committees, she worked to pass numerous bills to improve childcare and the educational system.

Early on in NAWHO's development, Patsy provided her support and helped establish NAWHO's credibility. She died in 2002, but while she was alive, she never turned down a request from us for help. I think that's truly rare for an elected official at her level. Patsy was always giving me challenges to further her cause. One of these was to organize a conference for Asian American women in political leadership, which I did in 1997.

At the time, there were very few Asian women in national political leadership positions. Patsy was the only Asian American woman in Congress. But there were more Asian American women serving at local levels, including mayors, school board, and city council members. We had two goals to accomplish with the 1997 summit—to get Asian American women elected officials to become health advocates for the community by teaching them more about our issues, and to build a network of Asian American women in elected office to provide support to one another and the next generation of leaders.

Another prominent Asian American political leader who provided inspiration and support as a participant in NAWHO's early work is Congressman Robert Matsui. Bob has served as a US representative from California for more than twenty years, and his goals on Capitol Hill have been closely aligned to those of NAWHO. He was instrumental in passing health insurance and welfare reforms that help children as well as securing $1 billion in funding for family preservation programs. Bob was also a proponent of the 1988 Civil Liberties Act that granted reparations for the former internees of Japanese American concentration camps in World War II.

Once NAWHO had its initial funding, I began to focus efforts to help the Asian American community and the health care system connect. Our first order of business was to gather and publish reliable and timely data on Asian American health. We did this through surveys and focus groups, and then used the data to influence improvements in public health programs. NAWHO also began to develop culturally appropriate community education and outreach programs and materials.

One of NAWHO's first projects was the South Asian Women's Health Project. At the time, no other Asian American community organizations were addressing this segment of the population. This project provided advocacy and public education to raise awareness of the health needs of this immigrant community. More than 150 South Asian women, a majority of whom did not have health insurance, participated in the health assessment that culminated in the first South Asian Women's Health Day. The program brought together more than a hundred low-income women from the community to discuss their health issues and concerns. Participants and other members of the South Asian community, who felt the importance of continuing to organize and discuss women's health issues, subsequently organized a similar event.

As additional funding became available, NAWHO also worked with health practitioners to tailor their services to the needs of their local Asian American communities, making them aware of Asian Americans' communication differences, cultural sensitivities, social practices, standards of privacy, and beliefs, and helping health care providers deal with Asian Americans in such a way that would allay fears and build trust.

The Asian Women's Reproductive and Sexual Health Empowerment Project conducted a health needs assessment of the factors influencing the use of reproductive and sexual health services by Asian American women. Reproductive health needs of Asian American women had been a priority from the time our work began since the issue of reproductive freedom is at the forefront of the promotion of gender equality.

Interviews and focus groups with Asian women of different ages as well as ethnic, immigration, and socioeconomic backgrounds revealed that Asian American women were not accessing reproductive health care services because they felt they were at low risk for breast and cervical cancers as well as sexually transmitted diseases. Cultural factors, such as the association of shame with talking about health issues—particularly sexual health issues—as well as a lack of access to information about sexual and reproductive health were some of the primary factors associated with the misperception of low risk.

Early on, NAWHO also addressed breast cancer in the Asian American community, conducting regional cultural competency training for health care providers that stressed the need to increase outreach and early detection services to immigrant Asian women. NAWHO also collected linguistically and culturally appropriate resources and information and served as a clearinghouse for Asian women with breast cancer, as well as for individuals and organizations interested in breast cancer among Asian women. In the area of policy development, NAWHO convened the first National Asian American Breast Cancer Summit, which brought together Asian community advocates and representatives from government health programs to create a plan of action that involved Asian American women in all levels of the fight against breast cancer.

In the first few years, NAWHO produced a number of needs assessment and research reports that provided policy and community recommendations on addressing the needs of this underserved population. These included *Perceptions of Risk: An Assessment of the Factors Influencing Use of Reproductive & Sexual Health Services by Asian American Women, Expanding Options: A Reproductive and Sexual Health Survey of Asian American Women,* and *Emerging Communities: A Health Needs Assessment of South Asian Women in Three California Counties.*

NAWHO also was working to build relationships with mainstream women's health and reproductive rights organizations in addition to health care organizations.

By 1995, NAWHO had information to share, and so, on November 17 and 18, we held our first conference with focus on breaking the silence surrounding Asian American women's health issues. The Mayor of San Francisco had declared the weekend Asian Women's Health Days, and I truly felt we were on the map. But as the conference approached, I had some fear that attendance wouldn't be what I'd expected. First then-President Bill Clinton and the GOP Congress disagreed over federal spending levels, causing a shutdown of the federal government. And then the weather didn't cooperate—there was a major fog problem impeding travel to California.

So, I was thrilled when three hundred people showed up at NAWHO's first conference. Until that time, I had never publicly shared the story of my sister. But since our theme was "breaking the silence," I decided that it was time I broke mine. In my address to attendees, I talked about my sister as an example of how the Asian American community lets culture and stigma prevent them from seeking health care.

I was really nervous about telling my story, and so I told it really fast, thinking that would make it easier. I was shaking the whole time. Afterwards, the number of people who came up to me and shared their own stories of losing a friend or a sister or a mother overwhelmed me.

That original conference was energizing, not only to me and to NAWHO, but I believe to the community as a whole. Interest in our work grew, and, by the time we held our second conference in 1997, "Coming Together, Moving Strong: Mobilizing an Asian Women's Health Movement," NAWHO had a staff—three others and myself! I was energized by this meeting, which was held in Los Angeles and brought 530 participants together to discuss issues that are often brushed aside in the greater Asian American community, such as domestic violence, young women's sexual health, breast cancer, and menopause. With the assistance of the California

Wellness Foundation, we were able to grant a hundred scholarships to low-income Asian women to attend.

In its first three years, NAWHO accomplished many "firsts." We implemented groundbreaking programs that initiated powerful organizing efforts at the grassroots level, involving Asian women and girls from different ethnic communities and across class lines. Our initial projects also assessed the health status of the diverse Asian women's community and created an advocacy and public policy framework that reflected commonalties and differences within the Asian community.

In 1998, we started a new effort to increase participation in public policy development nationwide. Congressman Matsui had often talked to me about the importance of becoming more active in the public policy arena. At the time NAWHO was founded, Patsy Mink was the only Asian American woman in either the US Senate or the House of Representatives. Furthermore, only eleven Asian American/Pacific Islander women sat in state legislatures—far below 1 percent of the total number of state legislators (7,424) in the United States—with no representatives in California, which has the largest population of Asian Americans in the country. In the advocacy arena, Asian American women in executive positions of leading mainstream nonprofit organizations (i.e., women's, civil rights, or health agencies) were few and far between.[5] So NAWHO began a new effort to increase the opportunities for Asian American women to become leaders in areas of decision-making on public policy that could effect the health care circumstances NAWHO was working to change.

Most leadership models at work at the time simply did not address advocacy and leadership development of Asian American women, particularly young women. Any existing programs focused purely on career advancement, rather than grassroots organizing, community development, or public health awareness. Thus, social justice efforts had suffered from the lack of participation of Asian American women who could make great contributions toward improving the welfare of the country. We believed that a change in societal values and the framework within which women's health is viewed required Asian American women to be given the opportunities to become equal and able leaders and join the concerted efforts of community members, health care providers, government officials, and the general population.

In order to change these conditions and improve the health status of Asian American communities, NAWHO began work to involve Asian American women at the national and local level in policy decisions about public health, and to promote strategic planning and action toward solving our nation's social problems. We started this process by reframing the discussion on women's health issues in this country to include Asian American and other women of color through various programs and collaborations. To further these efforts, NAWHO, with support from the W. K. Kellogg Foundation, began a leadership development program to greatly expand the leadership base of Asian American women, improving their skills in order to better organize both within their own communities and as a national body around health issues.

We called this effort the NAWHO National Leadership Network, which involved a broad range of emerging Asian American women leaders by facilitating communications, sponsoring skills-building training sessions, providing technical assistance, and delegating conference speakerships and other lead roles that call for the involvement of Asian American women. The National Leadership Network is an innovative project that has increased problem-solving skills and abilities among Asian American women, particularly for the underserved and underrepresented such as low-income, immigrant, and young women, who are often overlooked even within current Asian American leadership efforts. The National Leadership Network worked to instill a sense of self-empowerment among these women to encourage them to find solutions for health and social problems, shaping the future of their own lives and their communities.

The National Leadership Network brought one hundred emerging leaders to Washington, DC in 1998, 1999, and 2000 for a four-day training module. During the first two days, knowledgeable speakers from the Centers for Disease Control and Prevention and the National Institutes of Health provided participants with information about the status of Asian American health, including an overview of the most current research, model Asian American health programs and trends in health care. On the third day, participants experienced a White House briefing cosponsored by the Office of Women's Outreach at the White House where high-level speakers discussed policy issues as they related to Asian Americans. The fourth day was spent on Capitol Hill with official visits for all participants. The NAWHO staff and consultants helped to make appointments for each National Leadership Network participant with their particular members of Congress so that they could provide these elected officials with the latest information on Asian American women's health issues.

A highpoint of the training was a session with Congressman Robert Matsui, who talked to these dynamic women about taking a larger role in the political process—not only once a year but also every day in their own communities. Bob is a rare leader who brought this sense of urgency to me to push on to work for positive change. He challenged me and helped me to think differently and to expand NAWHO's coalition of supporters.

I also learned that our culture doesn't encourage Asian Americans to seek positions of political leadership. I found this out firsthand in a casual conversation one day with a doctor at the Chinatown Health Clinic in New York. After remarking that this doctor's parents must be proud of his accomplishments, I was surprised when he told me that he had really wanted to be a lawyer and to go into politics. However, his parents didn't think that politics was an honorable profession and told him he should pursue medicine instead.

1998 was a defining year for NAWHO. Not only did we make our presence known in Washington, DC with the National Leadership Network conference but also we received our first multimillion-dollar grant. Competing with hundreds of applicants, NAWHO was one of seven groups to win funding for the National Breast and Cervical Cancer Training & Replication Program from the Centers for Disease Control and Prevention. The grant of $2 million put NAWHO on the map for other major education grants dealing with specific issues—such as immunization—that are critical to Asian Americans.

Change comes slowly, but the Asian American movement has made great strides in the last decade. In 2000, NAWHO was part of a coalition that succeeded in advocating for a White House Executive Order on Asian Americans that mandated that all federal government programs must include Asian Americans in their data. This was only the second executive order in American history concerning Asians—the first concerned the internment of Japanese Americans during World War II.

I was proud to be a part of the group there to watch President Clinton sign the order, and I know that it has made a difference. Not only did the order establish a White House Office specifically for Asian American issues, but also a mandate for better data collection that will lead the way to more equitable distribution of funds not only for health programs but also housing, employment, and more.

Over the past ten years, NAWHO has grown to include four thousand members and supporters in twenty-five states and has secured more than $14 million in funding from some of the country's preeminent foundations and government agencies. NAWHO's strategic partnerships with public and private health organizations, businesses, and academic institutions have resulted in important research and education efforts that are shattering the myth of the model minority and building healthy futures for Asian Americans.

CHAPTER FIVE

Sitting in the Dark

The Asian American Osteoporosis Education Initiative

I have this vivid memory of my grandmother sitting in the dark. I was visiting Korea after my family had moved back there. I had been out with my brother and when I came home, I walked into the house, and my grandmother was sitting there in the dark living room.

"Halmughni, why didn't you turn on some lights?" I asked her.

She told me she couldn't turn on the lights because she couldn't reach the light switch.

My grandmother had broken her hip in a fall when she was in her seventies and she never walked again. She spent two decades crawling from room to room. She was completely disabled and completely accepting of it.

Years later, after I started NAWHO, I realized that many of the Asian American women on my staff and others I met had grandmothers with similar stories. All of our grandmothers were tiny little women with stooped shoulders. We thought that's just what Asian grandmothers looked like. We didn't know that they were literally shrinking as their spines weakened and fractured from osteoporosis.

Now, of course, I know that their condition was completely preventable. But that's only because I have been involved as an advocate for Asian American women's health. The information that crosses my desk is lost to the vast majority of Asian American women.

Recently I had my own bone density test and found that even though I'm only in my thirties, I'm at risk for osteoporosis. Like many Asians, my typical diet does not include milk and cheese products, so I usually don't get enough calcium or Vitamin D in my diet to help prevent osteoporosis. That's why, I've started taking supplements to avoid the disease that crippled my grandmother. And in the years ahead, I will continue to have bone density tests to measure the strength of my bones. This quick, painless noninvasive test is usually done on the hip, wrist, or spine or on the heel or hand. Women sixty-five and older even may be eligible for Medicare coverage of a bone mineral density test. It's a simple solution for a dangerous condition. But the vast majority of Asian American women are still sitting in the dark without the power of this knowledge.

Many Asian American women don't understand that osteoporosis can be deadly. Fractures of the spine can cause chronic pain, disfigurement, difficulty in breathing, and impaired movement. Hip fractures can be even more serious, resulting in permanent disabilities and even death. Twenty-four percent of hip-fracture patients age fifty and older will die within a year after a fracture.[1]

With diets low in calcium, body structures characterized by relatively low weight and small bones, and a tendency toward lactose intolerance, postmenopausal Asian American women have a disproportionately high risk for developing osteoporosis. According to the Office of Minority Health Resource Center, more than one fifth of Asian American women age fifty and older currently suffer from osteoporosis. Findings from a 1998 study by the National Osteoporosis Risk Assessment (NORA) found that 65 percent of postmenopausal Asian American women had low bone mineral density—the highest rate of all racial groups. The same NORA study also found that 8.2 percent of Asian American women with low bone mineral density had osteoporosis, compared to 5.2 percent of Caucasian women.[2]

Postmenopausal Asian American women are particularly at risk for developing osteoporosis because bone loss occurs more quickly in older age when the levels of estrogen, a hormone that protects bone density, have decreased. Also, it's estimated that as many as 90 percent of Asians suffer from lactose intolerance, which is a serious impediment to having a calcium rich diet that could counteract bone loss.[3]

Another risk factor contributing to the disparity is that many Asian Americans don't get enough exercise. For example, one national study found that 42 percent of Asian Americans did not engage in leisure-time physical activity.[4]

Because of the misperception that Asian Americans are statistically healthier than other minorities or Caucasians, important prevention messages are not reaching the community. Factors such as language barriers, low literacy, lack of orientation towards preventive care, lack of familiarity with Western health care systems, financial constraints, and transportation needs all stand between Asian American women and health information and services.

In response to this high risk of osteoporosis among Asian American women and communities, in 1999, NAWHO initiated a program to provide osteoporosis education to Asian American women. This one-time project in Sacramento, California included tailored Asian language health education seminars on osteoporosis that were implemented through collaborations with local, Asian American community-based organizations. An evaluation of these initial seminars demonstrated significant positive results among participants, including increased knowledge of osteoporosis as well as increased intentions to practice osteoporosis prevention.

So, following this successful demonstration, NAWHO developed *Living Healthy: The Asian American Osteoporosis Education Initiative.* Made possible with funding from the National Institutes of Health Osteoporosis and Related Bone Diseases-National Resource Center, the national initiative provides Asian women with the knowledge and resources to care for themselves and their families in a way that can reduce osteoporosis and lead to the improved health and well-being of Asian American women and their families.

Living Healthy seeks to fill the gap in culturally competent education on osteoporosis by achieving the following specific goals:

- ◆ Raising awareness of osteoporosis among postmenopausal Asian American women, including their risk factors for the disease, the diagnosis and treatment of the disease, and the consequences of the disease.
- ◆ Empowering postmenopausal Asian American women to prevent osteoporosis by engaging in positive lifestyle behaviors, such as sufficient calcium and vitamin D intake and exercise, and by consulting their doctors about the disease.

The central message of *Living Healthy* is that simple lifestyle changes can have profound impact on quality of life. Osteoporosis, a disease of poor bone health where bones become porous and weak, is not a normal part of aging, and can be prevented throughout one's lifetime by healthy bone behaviors.

The *Living Healthy* curriculum carries important messages, not only to older Asian American women but also to younger Asian Americans of both sexes, since the disease can also effect men. Healthy bone behaviors to prevent osteoporosis are important throughout life. In addition to diet and exercise, these include avoidance of cigarette smoking and excess alcohol. The sooner these habits are incorporated into day-to-day living, the better, but osteoporosis prevention can start at any age.

By acknowledging the caretaker role that Asian American women occupy in their families, the curriculum further extends its positive influence in the community. Explaining that activities that once were done without a second thought—such as bending over to pick up a newspaper or hug a grandchild—can cause a bone to break in people with osteoporosis is a powerful motivator. *Living Healthy* also includes information to help women who attend the sessions help their families. It explains that although older women are probably at highest risk for osteoporosis in the family, their husbands, children, and grandchildren are also at risk. The curriculum goes on to share information they need to know to help their family members reduce their risk.

Men:

- ♦ As men age, their risk for osteoporosis increases. One in every eight men over age fifty is at risk for having an osteoporotic fracture.[5] Each year, eighty thousand men suffer a hip fracture, and one-third of these men die within a year from complications.[6] Men also develop painful spinal fractures of osteoporosis, but usually at a later age than women do.
- ♦ Calcium deficiency, age-related loss of bone and muscle strength, low testosterone (male sex hormone) levels, long-term use of glucocorticoid medications, alcohol

abuse, smoking, and physical inactivity are causes of osteoporosis in men. If your partner suffers a bone fracture or loses height, ask him to talk to a doctor.
♦ Help your partner get enough calcium and vitamin D (he needs as much as you do) and plenty of physical activity to keep his bones and muscles strong.

Adult children:

♦ Good bone health practices are important for women and men at all ages. Adults, ages 19–50, should get 1000 mg/day of calcium, 400–800 IU/day of vitamin D, and plenty of weight-bearing and weight-resistance exercise. It is best to avoid smoking and excessive use of alcohol.
♦ Adults with inflammatory disorders such as rheumatoid arthritis, asthma, and lupus are at high risk for osteoporosis because their conditions are commonly treated with glucocorticoid medications that cause bone loss and fractures. People taking these medications should talk to their doctors about treatment that can minimize bone loss, but should *not* stop treatment or change the dose of their medications without consulting their physicians.
♦ If your daughter has experienced early menopause or a surgically induced menopause (removal of her ovaries), she will be at higher risk of bone loss and osteoporosis as a result.

Grandchildren:

♦ Osteoporosis prevention begins during the bone building years of childhood. About 85 percent to 90 percent of final adult bone mass is acquired by age eighteen in girls and age twenty in boys.[7] Children ages 4–8 should get 800 mg/day of calcium and children ages 9–18 should get 1300 mg/day. Vitamin D, weight bearing exercises, and the avoidance of smoking and alcohol will significantly reduce their risk of osteoporotic fractures later in life.

- Research suggests that Asian boys and girls have lower calcium intakes (35 percent), lower levels of physical activity (15 percent) and lower bone mineral density than their Caucasian counterparts.[8]
- Girls and boys who suffer from asthma and take glucocorticoid medications should be especially careful to practice good bone health habits that can help minimize the effects of the medication on their bone development.
- Teenaged girls also face special risks. Inadequate nutrition, which includes reduced calcium intake, reduced levels of physical activity, and diets leading to eating disorders, can lead young girls to become osteoporotic, experiencing spine and other fractures forty to fifty years before they otherwise would.[9]

Living Healthy structures practical information—like which foods contain calcium and vitamin D, exercise recommendations, and how to guard against falls—to best appeal to Asian Americans. The following helpful lists give older Asian American women an easy guide to prevent osteoporosis.

Where You Can Get Calcium
(1200 mg/day)

- Tofu
- Bok choy
- Broccoli
- Sardines with bones
- Salmon with bones
- Almonds
- Oysters
- Turnip leaves
- Seaweed (fresh)
- Napa cabbage
- Soybeans
- Milk
- Yogurt

- Cheese
- Ice cream
- Calcium-fortified orange juice
- Calcium-fortified soy milk
- Calcium-fortified rice

Where You Can Get Vitamin D
(400–800 IU/day)

- 10–15 minutes of sunshine
- Egg yolks
- Saltwater fish
- Liver
- Cod liver oil
- Vitamin D-fortified dairy and other food products

Types of Activities or Exercises to Do

- Take walks with grandchildren.
- Walk to grocery stores, shopping centers, or bus stops.
- Go on walks with friends.
- Take a ballroom dance class.
- Climb stairs, using handrails.
- Take pets on walks.
- Practice weight-resistance exercises (e.g., use soup cans as weights for lifting).

Examples of Balancing and Strengthening Exercises That Can Help Prevent You from Falling Too Easily

- Tai chi.
- While holding the back of a chair, the sink, or the counter top, practice standing on one leg at a time for one minute. Gradually, increase the time. If safe, try balancing with your eyes closed or without holding on.
- While holding the back of a chair, the sink, or the counter top, practice standing on your toes and then rock back to balance on your heels. Hold each position for a count of ten.

♦ While holding the back of a chair, the sink, or the counter top with both hands make a big circle to the left with hips, then repeat to the right. Do not move your shoulders or feet. Repeat five times.

Prevention Tactics for Home

♦ At home, wear slippers that have sturdy, nonslippery soles.

♦ Use nonskid mats near the sink and the stove in the kitchen.

♦ Make your home a safe place by putting things away, keeping floors smooth but not slippery, keeping areas well-lit, and keeping things you need in easy-to-reach areas.

♦ Use handrails when going up and down stairs.

Ways to Fall that Can Lessen Your Chance of Fracturing a Bone:

♦ Try to fall forward or to land on your buttocks. Falling sideways or straight down can more likely lead to a hip fracture.

♦ If possible, land on your hands or use objects around you to break the fall. You may fracture your wrist, but that is not as serious as a hip fracture.

NAWHO's latest osteoporosis education tool takes the *Living Healthy* curriculum to the next level. The *Living Healthy* Implementation Kit is a step-by-step instruction manual for planning, implementing, teaching, and evaluating a culturally competent osteoporosis seminar for postmenopausal Asian American women. Being tested by community-based partner organizations, the Implementation Kit is becoming a model program for raising awareness of osteoporosis among Asian American women and for empowering them to take action on the disease so that they no longer will have to sit in the dark.

CHAPTER SIX

Building Healthy Futures

The Global Movement against Tobacco

I was sixteen years old when I started smoking. I picked up a cigarette and immediately felt more like an American girl.

Almost all of the Korean American kids I hung out with smoked, boys and girls. My girlfriends and I thought it was liberating and sexy for women to smoke. We smoked those long, thin cigarettes that savvy marketers created just for us and envisioned ourselves similarly long and thin. Since smoking was still completely taboo for women in Korea, it made us feel rebellious and daring. Our parents certainly would have disapproved, and we hid it from them well.

Of course I had no idea at the time how addictive cigarettes were or how hard it would be for me to quit. I certainly was aware that smoking wasn't good for me. But I didn't understand that smoking was an identifying risk factor for many serious health problems such as lung cancer, cardiovascular disease, diabetes, asthma, and infant mortality.[1]

I wasn't thinking about any of those risks then—I was sixteen. The most important thing to me at the time was to fit in, to be like all of the other kids I knew, and to be

"American." In my view, smoking cigarettes helped me to achieve all of these.

A decade later, after many failed tries, I finally quit. I fully understood the health risks by then—and that I had been a perfect demographic fit for the cigarette marketing that was targeted toward females and Asian American teens. But what finally motivated me to quit was NAWHO. How could I be a successful advocate for women's health and smoke? I knew I had to quit, so I did. But truly it was one of the hardest things I've ever done.

When NAWHO officially joined the fight against tobacco, I began to learn that my experience with smoking was all too typical among Asian Americans. The Centers for Disease Control and Prevention (CDC) and the US surgeon general have released various reports on women and smoking and tobacco use among US racial minority groups, and the information is shocking.

In *Women and Smoking: A Report of the Surgeon General 2001*, US Surgeon General David Satcher, M.D., Ph.D., describes the problem in the strongest terms.

"When calling attention to public health problems, we must not misuse the word 'epidemic.' But there is no better word to describe the 600 percent increase since 1950 in women's death rates for lung cancer, a disease primarily caused by cigarette smoking," Satcher said. "Clearly, smoking-related disease among women is a full-blown epidemic."

The report outlines that more women become ill and die from smoking-related diseases than any other single cause and that tobacco use remains the leading cause of preventable deaths in the United States, accounting for more than 400,000 deaths each year.

The patterns apparent in the report's findings about cigarette usage and tobacco-related deaths make it clear why smoking is now a women's issue.

- In the 1990s, the decline in smoking rates among adult women stalled; at the same time, rates were rising steeply among teenage girls.
- Nearly all women who started smoking as teenagers and 30 percent of high school senior girls are still current smokers.
- In 2001 alone, lung cancer killed nearly 68,000 US women—27,000 more deaths than from breast cancer.
- In 1999, about 165,000 women died prematurely from smoking-related diseases like cancer and heart disease.
- Lung cancer is now the leading cause of cancer death among US women, with about 90 percent of all lung cancer deaths among women who continue to smoke being attributable to smoking.

The surgeon general's report also concluded that tobacco industry marketing was a major factor influencing girls to smoke in both the United States and overseas since tobacco ads and promotions targeted to women used themes of social desirability and independence. The report pointed out that women have been extensively targeted in tobacco marketing, including the development of brands specifically for women. Between 1995 and 1998, the report stated, expenditures for domestic cigarette advertising and promotion increased from $4.9 billion to $6.73 billion.

The report's findings about the perceptions of smoking among girls were startling. Not only do they perceive smoking to be "risk taking and rebelliousness," but also that smoking can control weight and negative moods. Also girls who smoke have less knowledge of the adverse consequences of smoking and overall have a positive image of smokers.

Among Asian American women, the surgeon general's report showed that smoking prevalence had decreased from 1979 through 1992, but then increased from 1995 through 1998. And from 1990 through 1994, smoking prevalence for high school senior girls was highest among American Indians (39 percent) and Caucasians (33 percent) followed by Hispanics (19.2 percent), Asian Americans (13.8 percent) and African Americans (8.5 percent).

The hopeful news, though, was that anti-smoking campaigns were making inroads. To work against tobacco marketing campaigns that equate success and empowerment for women with smoking, an aggressive, sustained anti-smoking program in California was praised in the report for influencing a decline in women's lung cancer rates there while rates continued to rise in the rest of the country.

These findings underscored the need for women's advocacy groups like NAWHO to aggressively continue efforts to educate their constituencies about the risks of smoking. NAWHO had been actively involved in the fight against tobacco since 1994 following a report by the National Center for Health Statistics, Centers for Disease Control and Prevention (CDC) that indicated Asian Americans were not an at-risk population because they had the lowest rate—13.9 percent—of cigarette smoking among all racial groups.[2]

Simply because of my own experiences, I wanted to look into this. Again, I was seeing that the myth of the model minority—Asians don't smoke; Asians are healthy—was putting the community at risk. Since many national studies as well as education and prevention dollars are based upon such attention-grabbing statistics, I knew that Asian American communities would lose out on critically needed public health programs. How could usage be so low when I knew that Koreans and many other Asian ethnic groups still thought that cartons of cigarettes were acceptable gifts for birthdays and holidays? Members of my family were certainly still following this practice.

Upon a closer look, we found that the CDC surveys had been conducted in English, by phone, and had used only a small sample. Since English is not the first language of so many Asian immigrants, we knew that the numbers must not be representative.

With $75,000 in funding from Kaiser Permanente - California Division and the National Home Office of the American Cancer Society, NAWHO developed a survey utilizing the same tobacco-use questions from the CDC study with one key difference: those questions were translated into native languages for Korean and Vietnamese to reach two of the largest Asian American ethnic groups in the United States. This survey became the first national, multi-lingual assessment to measure tobacco use and exposure among Vietnamese and Korean American men and women.

NAWHO commissioned Interviewing Services of America (ISA), a national market research firm specializing in multi-lingual, Asian-specific research, to administer and translate the survey as well as to compile and analyze the data.

We also took great care to ensure that ISA selected a sample that would accurately reflect these two segments of the Asian American population. The sample included two hundred Vietnamese American men, two hundred Vietnamese American women, two hundred Korean American men and 211 Korean American women ages eighteen and over. They were selected randomly based on Asian surnames from the Donnelly DQ2 People Bank that contained 85 million households with telephones in the United States. And the geographic distribution of those chosen for the survey closely followed that of the 1990 US Census.

The surveys were conducted from December 1997 to January 1998 using professional bilingual interviewers who surveyed each respondent in their preferred language— either English or their native language.

Every effort was made to ensure the integrity of the survey; however, it certainly didn't claim to represent all Asian Americans—or even all Vietnamese Americans or Korean Americans. Our sample didn't include Asian Americans without telephones or those without Asian surnames. But the NAWHO survey's findings were so significantly different from those of the CDC survey, that we believe it provided keen insight into the health status of Asian Americans. Further, and most importantly, the NAWHO report, *Smoking Among Asian Americans: A National Tobacco Survey*, laid the groundwork for a number of effective tobacco control programs.

Smoking Among Asian Americans: A National Tobacco Survey found that Asian American men were smoking at much higher rates than were being reported by the federal government and were, therefore, at a much higher risk for tobacco-related diseases and health problems than was previously thought. It showed that 34 percent of Vietnamese and 31 percent of Korean American men in the survey currently smoked compared to the rate for Asian American men of 20 percent that had been previously reported. According to the NAWHO survey, smoking prevalence among Asian American men was much higher than that of Caucasian men, who had a reported rate of 28 percent.

Smoking Among Asian Americans: A National Tobacco Survey also found that Asian American women were at extremely high risk for tobacco-related health problems from second hand smoke, both at home and in the workplace.

Thirty-six percent of both Vietnamese and Korean American women reported living in a household with one or more smokers; and 31 percent of Vietnamese and 27 percent of Korean American women said they were exposed to second hand smoke at home every day. Compounding their risk was the fact that 41 percent of Korean and 27 percent of Vietnamese American women who worked said they were exposed to second hand smoke at the workplace every day.

This data helped to explain the high rate of lung cancer among Asian American women. Even while a relatively low number of Asian American women smoke, lung cancer is the leading cause of preventable death among Asian American women over the age of fifty-five.

The NAWHO report showed that Asian American smokers started smoking at a young age and continued to smoke heavily into adulthood. In fact, 52 percent of Vietnamese and 33 percent of Korean Americans who smoked said they tried their first cigarette at eighteen years old or younger. Of those who still smoked, 82 percent said they smoked every day as opposed to just some days. And 35 percent of smokers said they smoked at least one pack a day, and more than two-thirds said they had tried to quit and failed.

These statistics alone showed that the marketing aimed at Asian American youth was working all too well.

The numbers revealed that tobacco education programs were not reaching Asian Americans with vital information about the harmful effects of smoking. Approximately one in five Vietnamese and Korean Americans said they did not know that smoking caused heart disease, bronchitis, emphysema, chronic obstructive pulmonary disease, and mouth cancer.

A surprising 34 percent of Vietnamese Americans surveyed said they didn't know that smoking tobacco was addictive. And even though Asian Americans have extremely low rates of utilizing preventive clinical services, half of those who had visited a health care professional were not being asked about their smoking habits or educated about the risks of smoking during routine physical exams. This fact alone indicated that the misperception that Asian Americans do not smoke had impeded valuable opportunities for education.

Perhaps the most important result of the NAWHO study was its clear illustration that data collection methods then being used by national surveys were inadequate and were not reaching underserved Asian Americans. By translating survey questions into native languages, NAWHO was able to reach a broader sample and improve the quality of the collected data. Almost all respondents—99 percent of Vietnamese and 94 percent of Korean Americans—surveyed were born outside of the United States. Most of them—89 percent of Vietnamese and 82 percent of Korean Americans— requested to be surveyed in their native language. As a result, this methodology was able to show that smoking was a far more serious problem among Asian Americans than had previously been reported.

Further, the NAWHO report showed that in order for tobacco control and public health intervention programs to successfully reach the Asian American community, they needed to specifically target Asian American women and girls. Because Asian American women are at the center of health and social service coordination in their communities, involving women in future tobacco control programs emerged as a priority. Given the high prevalence of second hand smoke exposure in the home and the lack of knowledge of the comprehensive health risks associated with smoking, NAWHO called for programs that would target Asian American women and girls with the latest information about the risks of smoking, such as the dangers of combining the use of birth control pills and smoking due to strong links to heart disease and stroke.

Of course we knew one study was not enough. Because of the great diversity within the Asian American community, we recommended further studies targeting Asian American subpopulations such as Laotians and Filipinos as well as studies targeting teens to help prevention programs make a greater impact.

NAWHO launched a cooperative agreement with the CDC Office on Smoking in 1998. The partnership was designed to collect additional information within the Asian American community, which included immigrants from more than thirty countries aligned with the most recent US Census, and to educate our own community leaders about the harmful impact of smoking on women's health. One of these studies targeted an especially high-risk group— Southeast Asian youth

From April though May of 2000, NAWHO surveyed 708 Southeast Asian youth between the ages of thirteen and eighteen. To administer the surveys, NAWHO partnered with two community-based health organizations in California and Texas, where the majority of Southeast Asian Americans live. The East Dallas Counseling Center in Dallas, Texas and the Khmer Society of Fresno in Fresno, California conducted the surveys at a number of venues including Cambodian New Year celebrations, events at Laotian and Cambodian temples, local health and wellness events, cultural youth clubs and groups, and ethnic language schools. Although the methodology was using a convenient sample, this study provided important information about Southeast Asian youth.

What emerged was an insightful glimpse into tobacco use and exposure in these communities to help NAWHO and other organizations better target education and prevention campaigns. NAWHO found that almost 25 percent of the boys surveyed had tried smoking while just over 10 percent of the girls had. The majority of those who smoked began smoking between the ages of ten and fourteen. Most of the smokers got their cigarettes from peers (34 percent) or family members (27 percent), while others bought cigarettes from grocery stores (20 percent) or liquor stores (13 percent). Only 3 percent of those surveyed said that lack of access to cigarettes was an influence for not smoking. Instead, when asked why they smoked, 37 percent said friends and 29 percent said that family members had influenced their decision to smoke.

Confirming the need for a targeted prevention campaign was the fact that the respondents who did not smoke said their number one reason for not smoking was that it was detrimental to their health. Another 29 percent said they didn't smoke because their parents and family didn't approve.

Key findings confirmed that Southeast Asian youth were not aware of the serious health risks associated with smoking and had been significantly influenced by tobacco marketing in their countries of origin that glamorized smoking. This marketing is largely credited with the increase of smoking rates in Asian countries even while rates decrease in the United States and other Western countries. At the time of NAWHO's Southeast Asian youth study, an estimated three-quarters of the Asian American and Pacific Islander population in the United States was foreign born, bringing with them attitudes about smoking formed in those countries.[3]

NAWHO and other groups continue to advocate efforts that will reduce smoking among women. Additional research is needed to better understand and reduce current disparities in smoking prevalence among Asian women of different subgroups. There's little research on smoking cessation among

Asian women, so we must encourage the reporting of gen-der-specific results from studies of influences on smoking behavior and smoking prevention.

There is also work to be done to increase awareness of the impact of smoking on women's health. It's critical to take a broad-based approach to tobacco control, and address the larger socioeconomic factors and co-occurring health issues that shape smoking behaviors in underserved communities. No single factor determines patterns of tobacco use among Asian Americans. Instead these patterns are the result of complex interactions of multiple factors, such as socioeco-nomic status, cultural characteristics, and the process of learning the tradition of new culture once these immigrants reach the United States.

Taking a lesson from the success of the widespread, uni-fied effort to reduce breast cancer, we must continue to work to call public attention to the human and monetary costs of lung cancer and other smoking-related diseases. Tobacco use is not just an individual problem—it's a public health prob-lem that impacts the larger community. We must educate our business leaders, community leaders, and other stakeholders about this growing public health burden. Estimates show that smoking caused more than $150 billion in annual health-related economic loses from 1995 to 1999, including $81.9 billion in mortality-related productivity losses and $75.5 bil-lion in excess medical expenditures in 1998.[4]

To accomplish this, we need to encourage greater in-volvement of Asian American women and men in the fight against tobacco and continue to increase leadership opportu-nities for underserved populations through efforts such as the NAWHO National Leadership Network.

CHAPTER SEVEN

Organizing for Survival

The Truth about Breast
And Cervical Cancers

Wife, mother, caretaker, sister, grandmother—these are all acceptable roles for women in traditional Asian communities. And if women are subservient and obedient, adhere to tradition, and take on heavy domestic responsibilities—putting everyone before themselves—then they're worthy of great praise.

So why should we be surprised when a sixty-year-old Chinese American woman in Chicago who has breast cancer drinks bleach trying to kill herself so that she won't be a burden on her family? This woman's tragic story is consistent with a culture that discourages women from thinking of themselves before others.

Though there has been a movement within the Asian American community since the late 1960s to speak out for progress, the Asian immigrant community is still largely influenced by traditional values and isolated by language and economic barriers from seeking vital health care information and services. Second generation Asian Americans also find that the old ways and conflicts with their immigrant parents prevent them from pursuing their personal goals and interests. As a result, these traditional values are influencing both the physical and mental health of Asian Americans and threatening the well being of the community.

One of the solutions is to empower Asian Americans, particularly women, to make decisions and take action for their own health and well being. At the core of that empowerment effort is the effective dissemination of accurate health and prevention information.

Over the last decade, one of NAWHO's most capable spokespersons for organizing for positive community change has been Robin Chin. I first met Robin in 1997 when she came to NAWHO's National Leadership Network conference in Washington, DC. At the time, she was volunteering for the American Cancer Society. Robin, who is a breast cancer survivor, has helped me—and many others—understand what Asian American women go through when they are diagnosed with cancer.

Robin has a quiet but potent presence and tells her story with great dignity. When she first found out that she had cancer, she couldn't bring herself to share the news with her parents. Like so many Asian American women, she was shocked by her diagnosis because the general perception is that Asian women don't get breast cancer. She knew that her parents would certainly think that her cancer was fatal, so she didn't want to burden them with the news.

Instead of talking about her condition, Robin started a lonely search for information, treatment options, and statistics about breast cancer and Asian American women. Unfortunately the only research material she found was for Caucasian or African American women.

Robin understands why Asian American women think that a cancer diagnosis is a death sentence. But she's lived past that stigma and is now a living, breathing testament to the truth—it doesn't have to be. During the six years that Robin served as chair of the NAWHO Board of Directors, she shared her story countless times. Today she continues to lead by example, educating Asian American women to take responsibility for their own health care.

Central to the important message of intervention and prevention is getting the word out that Asian American women *do* get breast and cervical cancer. In Asia, women have some of the lowest incidence rates in the world for breast and cervical cancers. But when they migrate to the United States, the risk for these cancers increases six fold. Some studies show as high as an 80 percent greater risk for the disease among Asian American women in the United States compared to their counterparts in Asia.

The risk for some Asian women is extremely high. Vietnamese American women, for instance, have the highest rate of cervical cancer in the country. According to the National Cancer Institute, Vietnamese American women have cervical cancer rates of 43 cases per 100,000 women, which is almost three times higher than the next group, Latina women, who exhibit 17.1 cases per 100,000.[1]

Other Southeast Asian women are also showing high cervical cancer rates. In California, for instance, cervical cancer is the most common form of cancer among Laotian women and the second most common cancer for Cambodian American women.[2]

Perhaps the most disturbing trend is that while cervical cancer incidence rates for all other major racial groups in the United States have fallen in recent years, rates of cervical cancer among Asian American women alone are rising.[3]

Cervical cancer is one of the most preventable and curable diseases affecting women worldwide, but only when women get regular Pap smears that can identify precancerous conditions, targeting them for treatment before the disease fully develops. Certainly one contributing factor to these high incidence rates is the fact that less than half of Asian women over the age of fifty have had a clinical breast examination and mammogram within the past two years—the lowest screening rate among all women.

In partnership with the Centers for Disease Control and Prevention (CDC), NAWHO has mounted large-scale education and training efforts with the mission to eliminate these breast and cervical cancer health disparities among Asian American women. This effort came directly from NAWHO's constituency as participants at its first national conference, *Coming Together, Moving Strong: Mobilizing an Asian Women's Health Movement,* held in 1995, voiced their concern about the obvious Asian American void in the growing nationwide fight against breast cancer. In response to this powerful appeal by Asian American breast cancer survivors, community advocates, and health care providers, NAWHO began an innovative and unique series of initiatives to address these cancers at the community, medical, and policy levels.

We began with public education efforts to increase Asian American women's knowledge of breast and cervical cancers and available screening programs. We also started to build strong partnerships with breast cancer advocacy groups, becoming the only Asian American organization ever to serve on the board of the National Breast Cancer Coalition, a coalition that includes 55,000 individual and 450 organizational members.

To further build a presence for Asian Americans in the cancer movement and influence public policy, NAWHO

convened the first National Asian American Breast Cancer
Summit in New York City and its Follow-Up Meeting in
Napa, California in 1996. Through these meetings,
NAWHO brought together leaders in the breast cancer
field, including Asian American community advocates and
breast cancer survivors, women's health advocates, and
private industry and state and federal public health program representatives. Participants at this groundbreaking
summit identified four priority issues.

- ♦ Addressing gaps in research and data on breast cancer
  and Asian American women
- ♦ Ensuring culturally and linguistically competent outreach and early detection programs for Asian American
  women
- ♦ Improving accessibility of treatment programs for Asian
  American women, and
- ♦ Increasing the involvement of the Asian American community in the nationwide effort to combat cancer.

As a result of these two meetings, NAWHO published the
nation's only *National Plan of Action on Asian American
Women and Breast Cancer* that provided the first comprehensive recommendations in areas of technology, education, and
collaboration to impact the underserved Asian American
community. NAWHO officially unveiled this document to the
nation at a congressional briefing in Washington, DC cosponsored by the American Cancer Society. The briefing featured
congressional members Nancy Pelosi, Anna Eshoo, Patsy
Mink, and Louise Slaughter, who spoke to the crowd of more
than a hundred Capitol Hill staffers and federal agency representatives about making Asian American women a priority in
all levels of breast cancer advocacy. Since then, more than six
thousand copies of this action plan have been distributed to
all sectors involved in cancer control and community health.

With such tremendous success and proven capacity to raise awareness, build coalitions, and provide education and training, in September of 1997, NAWHO launched a five-year partnership with the CDC and eight state government health departments. This new program, *Communicating Across Boundaries*, began operating in conjunction with the National Breast and Cervical Cancer Early Detection Program, a CDC-funded initiative to provide free or low cost mammograms and Pap tests, as well as necessary diagnostic and follow-up services, to priority populations including older women, women with low incomes, and women of racial or ethnic minority groups. *Communicating Across Boundaries* has worked directly with state affiliates of this national program to increase the utilization of screening services by Asian American women. To accomplish this goal, *Communicating Across Boundaries* seeks specifically to:

♦ Promote responsiveness to the needs and views of Asian American women related to early detection screening by building the cultural competency of health care providers.
♦ Enhance the capacity of state and local breast and cervical cancer programs to provide outreach and screening services that are responsive to the needs and views of Asian American women.
♦ Provide public education on Asian American women and breast and cervical cancers to promote responsiveness to early detection screening in Asian American communities and the general public.
♦ Create sustainable and systematic collaborations between national, state, and local breast and cervical cancer providers and programs focused on improving the breast and cervical health of Asian American women.

We knew that we not only had to reach women in the community, but also health care providers. If providers were not aware of the risks Asian American women faced for breast and cervical cancer, then they might not initiate discussions about prevention and screening. Consider the all-too-common story of a thirty-six-year-old Japanese American woman with breast cancer. She said that after finding a lump in her breast, her doctor told her not to worry because Japanese women didn't get breast cancer.

The *Communicating Across Boundaries* curriculum contains the messages and skills-building exercises necessary for improved cultural competency with Asian American women. Using a model forged by the Division of Cancer Prevention and Control (DCPC) at the CDC, the curriculum was developed using a strict process of evidenced-based evaluation, pilot testing, and peer review in diverse geographic areas and with diverse groups of health care professionals.

The curriculum and training gives health care workers vital information about the attitudes, beliefs, and behaviors held by many Asian American women and how those effect health care. It also provides a full discussion of the concept of cultural competency to set the stage for progress.

What is Cultural Competency?

Cultural competency refers to the continually developing ability to respond to individuals of different cultures in a way that is sensitive to and respectful of the differences that exist between cultures. In a health care setting, this requires providers to be aware of the cultural values and beliefs of clients and to understand how these factors influence their health-seeking attitudes and behavior.

The importance of understanding the meaning of cultural competency is key to the development of cultural competency in the successful provision of breast and cervical cancer screening services to Asian American women. The ability to respond to clients in a sensitive, knowledgeable, and respectful manner creates an interaction that can be immensely more effective and well received, and that contributes to improved quality of care and long-term breast and cervical health.

Cultural competency, however, involves multiple factors that must continually improve over time. Too often, being culturally competent is understood to be a circumscribed set of actions or abilities, whereas the process of developing cultural competency is an ongoing learning experience. Understanding contributing factors to cultural competency and recognizing the ever-evolving nature of its development are crucial for continued improvement to occur.

There are a number of common factors among all definitions of cultural competency, including:

- Knowledge of cultural diversity and difference.
- Attitudes that accept and value cultural difference.
- Ability to communicate and respond to individuals of different cultures.
- Commitment to furthering understanding and knowledge of different cultures.

Necessary components for cultural competency in a health care setting include:

- Understanding that culture affects health knowledge, attitudes, beliefs, behaviors, and outcomes, and
- Commitment to addressing these influential cultural variables in the health care setting.

The NAWHO definition of cultural competency in the provision of breast and cervical cancer services to Asian American women recognizes that this is a process of behavioral change where health care providers develop and expand their knowledge of, sensitivity to, communication with, respect for, and capacity to reach individuals from Asian American communities who are shaped by a variety of histories, cultures, languages, religions, economic conditions, social and gender roles, and health practices and beliefs. Cultural competency in this sense may involve additional challenges related to the unique perceptions, needs, and fears of Asian American women surrounding these diseases. NAWHO defines a culturally competent breast and cervical cancer service provider to Asian American women as one who exhibits the following characteristics.

- Knowledge of breast and cervical cancers for Asian American women including statistics and the impact of immigration and other cultural factors on these data
- Awareness of the institutional, community, and provider level barriers Asian American women may face in seeking breast and cervical cancer early detection screening services
- Awareness of and practice with effective, sensitive, and open communication with Asian American women
- Familiarity with outreach strategies to recruit Asian Americans that are appropriately tailored to the needs of Asian American communities
- Knowledge of model education, outreach, or screening programs that exhibit cultural competency and innovative service-delivery to Asian American women
- Commitment to furthering Asian American women's understanding and knowledge of the influences of culture on health

The result of the process should be an environment for providing breast and cervical cancer early detection screening services that addresses Asian American women's awareness and fears, respects Asian American women's needs and barriers, and empowers Asian American women to take control of their own health care. Moreover, this environment should help breast and cervical cancer service providers to more effectively educate, recruit, and retain Asian American women for these essential services.[4]

Cultural competency can be understood as a continuum of competence levels or stages including:

Awareness. The individual or organization understands and acknowledges that cultural differences exist and impact health care and health delivery experiences.

Sensitivity. The individual or organization responds to cultural differences and attempts to take them into consideration as they provide health care services.

Knowledge. The individual or organization exhibits comprehensive knowledge and understanding about specific cultural norms, values, and beliefs, particularly those that impact their health care experiences.

Adaptability. The individual or organization utilizes the knowledge of the cultural norms, values, and beliefs to negotiate interactions successfully.

Competency. The individual or organization displays acceptance of and respect for cultural norms, values, and beliefs, and continually strives to gain and incorporate further understanding of the culture into their service systems and abilities.[5]

Once the curriculum sets the stage, it provides participants with an understanding of the beliefs shared by several Asian American communities as they relate to their responsibilities, relationships, health, and families to help providers negotiate health care situations by increasing their understanding of the perspectives Asian American women may hold as they enter the health care system. This helps providers identify their own misperceptions about these women and provides them with information needed to help correct them.

Because of the large number of Asian American ethnicities, cultures, and languages, we should take caution when describing all Asian American ethnic groups collectively. While common themes and belief systems seem to be present in most Asian American populations, variances exist not only among cultures but also among subgroups and families within one culture. With more than forty ethnic groups represented by the term "Asian and Pacific Islander," differences among cultures undoubtedly exist.

Laotians, for instance, believe that karma, or fate, drives them to continually strive for a state of spiritual liberation by ridding themselves of all earthly desires. Animism, which is the belief that spirits exist in natural objects or phenomena such as the wind or the lake, is also popular among Laotians. And since religion is so important in their lives, Laotians tend to understand causes of their illnesses through religious beliefs. The three most common theories used to explain the cause of disease are:

Naturalistic theory—Either "bad wind" or spoiled food is to blame.

Supernaturalistic theory—Disease and illness results from the influence of ancestral spirits, gods, demons, spirits, or malevolent spells.

Metaphysical theory—Imbalance within the "hot and cold" causes disease, similar to the Taoist yin and yang.

Regardless of whether they adhere to the naturalistic, supernaturalistic, or metaphysical theory, most Laotians believe that the primary cause of illness or disease may be attributed to the loss of one of the thirty-two spirits thought to inhabit the body and maintain health. The soul may be lost due to being startled when walking alone, having an accident, after travel, or other causes, and may be recalled through a soul-calling ceremony performed by a healer. As a protective measure, Laotians may wear a string tied around their wrists. They may also wear a talisman called *katha*, which is a string passed through a small cylinder of gold or brass that is inscribed with prayers. The curriculum instructs health providers that they should ask for the patient's consent before removing such articles.

This example—and many others included in the curriculum—provide important information about the traditional methods of treatment sought by various Asian cultures that is invaluable to health care workers if they are going to be able to provide successful outreach and treatment in the Asian American community.

While the curriculum cautions against generalization and provides many details about specific cultures, there are a number of traditional philosophical values and beliefs that are held by Asian Americans. These values and beliefs are based on long-standing Asian traditions, to which Asian Americans have often continued to adhere.

The following information offers an overview of the traditional philosophical values and beliefs that can be held by Asian Americans, focusing primarily on the Asian American cultures most prominent in the United States. While this information is loosely descriptive, it does not capture the specific beliefs held by all Asian American groups. Instead, the best strategy for providing breast and cervical cancer services to Asian American women involves discovering the specific beliefs held by the client and continually striving to avoid generalization.

Impact of Acculturation

Not only do Asian Americans represent a diverse set of ethnic and cultural backgrounds, but their life experiences and immigration histories may range broadly, as well. Individuals can be new immigrants with little exposure to American life-styles, but they can also be third, fourth, or fifth generation immigrants mentally, emotionally, and culturally bound to life in the United States. The level of their acculturation can dramatically influence their belief systems and their experiences with linguistic and cultural difference they face on a daily basis. Likewise, acculturation can affect their utilization of and response to the health care system, and providers should consider this factor in their interactions with their Asian American clients. To document the extent to which Asian American values can differ from those held in the United States, the information provided in this section reflects less-acculturated belief systems. Because individuals will vary in their level of acculturation, as well as in their specific cultural beliefs, training participants should not assume that all Asian American clients will exhibit the beliefs outlined below and instead seek to identify the particular beliefs their clients hold.

Asian American philosophical values and beliefs may differ markedly from those otherwise found in the United States. These values and beliefs are based on long-standing Asian traditions, to which Asian Americans have often continued to adhere. The following present several examples of traditional Asian values and beliefs that continue to influence Asian Americans in their daily lives and in their health seeking and receiving behaviors after they come to the United States. These "Asian" characteristics refer to Asians in their home countries before they have been influenced by American culture, thus the distinction in the text and use of "Asian" versus "Asian American."

Self-Concept

Asians often have a collective or interdependent self-conceptualization, meaning they view themselves as part of a larger group and have a strong sense of group loyalty. They may place significance on the ability to fulfill obligations and responsibilities based on a prescribed role within their group system. In addition, they often value group harmony over individual expression and derive self-esteem from their ability to further the goals of the group.

Family

The family is the primary group to which Asian individuals traditionally adhere. Asians often hold a strong sense of duty. Maintaining an honorable family reputation is highly prioritized. In addition, the needs of the family are typically placed above the needs of the individual. Many Asian individuals will involve their whole family in the decision-making process.

This sense of responsibility often keeps Asian Americans from seeking care. Consider the situation of a forty-five-year-old woman who had never had a mammogram even though she had insurance through her husband's employer. She also had never considered touching her breasts to exam them for lumps. She always had small breasts and thought there was no need for concern. When she began to feel some pressure in her left breast, she ignored it. When her left breast became swollen, she asked her husband what she should do. He told her to ignore it. When her breast became painful, and she was too tired to care for her children, she finally saw a doctor and was diagnosed with late-stage cancer. Still this woman did not tell anyone outside of her immediate family that she had cancer because she was afraid that the women in her church would gossip that she got cancer because she put herself before her family.

Gender Roles

Asian women are often taught to be obedient, respectful, and yielding. Women hold traditional duties of mothering and housekeeping, and defer to male authority figures in their decision-making. Women derive their value from their husband's families and from their ability to fulfill their prescribed responsibilities.

Social Interactions

Asians traditionally place importance on hierarchical familial and social relationships. A great deal of attention is given to role fulfillment within the culturally determined hierarchy. In addition, Asians can hold a strong sense of obligation and need for reciprocity, but also an aversion to assuming unnecessary obligation. Moreover, they often emphasize appropriate behavior and conduct, or a need to "save face," and demonstrate a corresponding tendency toward approval-seeking behavior.

Asian American Approaches to Health Care

Asian American approaches to health care may differ markedly from those otherwise found in the United States. Following are several examples of traditional Asian approaches to health care:

Attitudes toward General Health

Asians may have varying attitudes toward health and its origin. Health may be a function of destiny, chance, good fortune, strong will, divine intervention, or moral righteousness, for example. Traditional concepts of health, however, have not typically focused on empirical evidence.

Attitudes toward Illness and Death

Asians may believe that illness and death are part of the normal life cycle. Both are often believed to be due to destiny, bad luck, lack of will, or former misdeeds. As a result of these beliefs, Asians may be more likely to simply accept their illness or attempt to utilize alternative therapies rather than seek clinical treatments. Also, certain diseases are also considered disgraceful or shameful, which may discourage them from seeking treatment.

Attitudes toward the "Sick Role"

Asians may often display serenity or stoicism, and often take a heroic, self-healing approach to illness. In addition, pain is to be denied or tolerated as a sign of strength. Being sick can force one to be dependent, leading to feelings of helplessness, denial, or depression.

Attitudes toward Preventive Health

Asians often practice preventive health through the regulation of diet and exercise, and through the use of traditional medicines. When seeking medical help, however, they may wait until critical signs of illness or trouble arise to be treated. In addition, individuals' denial or silent tolerance of health problems can result in delayed health care access. For women, in particular, reproductive health care is often sought only with respect to pregnancy or family planning, and Asian women may not consider reproductive health care necessary in the absence of sexual activity.

Consider the case of a sixty-year old Chinese American woman who had recently immigrated to the United States to live with her adult son and his family. She had noticed changes in her breast but was afraid to ask her son to take her to a doctor because she didn't want to be a burden. Instead she applied herbal ointments to her breasts for a year. Only after she noticed abnormal discharges from both of her breasts and soreness in her left breast, and had discussed her pain with her elderly in-laws did she finally decide to seek medical help.

Attitudes toward Health Information

Asians may not always want to hear all the information available to them, particularly as it relates to their health and well being. Some Asian cultures, for example, believe that talking about the problem actually induces the ailment.

Attitudes toward Patient/Provider Interaction

Asians tend to respect the physician and place great value on the physician's recommendations. The physician is esteemed as having great virtue and is believed to be concerned, giving, and responsible for the patient's welfare. The patient is expected to show respect and deference for the physician's authority and is also expected to be grateful for the physician's services. Asians often view physicians as authority figures and may accept what they say without question, even when they may not understand what they are being told to do.

Attitudes toward Modern Treatments

Many Asians believe that modern American medicine is too strong for their Asian bodies. This may lead to their noncompliance for drug usage. In addition, Asian Americans may often rely on traditional remedies and utilize them in conjunction with prescription drugs.

One fifty-three-year-old Asian American woman had regular mammograms until the garment factory she worked for shut down. Without insurance, however, she could no longer afford the hospital visits. Instead, she increased her use of coin rubbing and herbs, traditional healing practices that she believed had protected her family for generations. Despite these efforts, she developed a high fever one day and decided to seek medical care. When she went to the clinic, the doctor seemed rushed and used several terms that she did not understand. She also felt that the doctor stared strangely where she had used her coins. After being examined, she considered asking the doctor about a mammogram, but changed her mind. Since the doctor did not mention it, she didn't think she should.

Women's Attitudes toward Bodies and Sexuality

Asian women can be uncomfortable with their own bodies and with their sexuality. They may exhibit modesty, even in health care settings, and are often uncomfortable with male physicians. Many believe that only their husbands should be concerned with their sexual experience or be familiar with their reproductive organs. Being curious or knowledgeable about the body is often considered inappropriate. For unmarried women, even talking about sexuality is often discouraged.

Moreover, Asian women may view their breasts only in terms of their function in breast-feeding.

Such was the case of one twenty-five-year old single woman who had never had a pelvic examination. She thought that if she was not married, then there was no need for such a procedure. Even then, she thought, who should be touching her body other than a husband? When she heard that a woman in her neighborhood was diagnosed with cervical cancer, she was shocked. Vietnamese women do not get cancer, she thought, but it did make her think about getting checked just in case. She considered going to the family planning clinic in her neighborhood, but changed her mind. The last time she went to a doctor, she had to wait for over an hour to be seen and nobody could understand her. Even the magazines in the waiting room were all in English.

Asian and American Communication Styles

It is also essential for health care providers to understand Asian communication styles, including the use of nonverbal modes of expression such as hand gestures, facial expressions, eye contact, and body language that may be subtle or indirect. Expressions of emotions such as fear or love are often conducted indirectly through actions rather than through words. Negative emotions, in particular, may be purposely suppressed in order to appear stoic. Expressions of positive emotions may be curtailed to project modesty.

American communication styles tend to use verbal modes of expression such as talking, laughing, and responding with verbal cues. Expressions of positive emotions such as love or happiness are expected, whereas expressions of negative emotions such as fear or sadness may be suppressed. The ability to articulate thoughts and emotions is highly valued as an indication of confidence and intelligence. Asking questions is considered a sign of interest rather than rudeness as it is in many Asian cultures.

These differing communication styles have great influence in the health care service delivery:

Verbalization

Health care service delivery in most American medical settings relies on patient verbalization. Patients are expected to verbalize their medical needs and concerns, and health care providers often depend on such information to diagnose and prescribe appropriately. Because Asian communication styles prioritize nonverbal modes of expression, the process of articulating medical needs and concerns may be unfamiliar and uncomfortable for many Asian American women patients. If language barriers are present, Asian American women may be unable to describe their medical needs and concerns so that a health care provider can understand them.

Directness

Because information is critical for accurate diagnosis, consent, and compliance, health care providers in most American medical settings may ask patients explicit questions about their health. Health care providers may also inquire directly about a patient's understanding of a medical procedure or outcome. Because Asian communication styles often rely on indirect modes of expression, answering direct questions about medical needs and concerns may feel uncomfortable and invasive to Asian American women patients. Because Asian American women may use indirect or subtle indications of understanding such as facial expressions or body language, health care providers may feel uncertain about a patient's comprehension of the medical situation being discussed.

Disclosure

Again, health care providers in most American medical settings rely on self-disclosed health information from patients in order to provide services. Protected by strict privacy regulations, the health care setting is often considered a safe environment for disclosing confidential personal information. Because Asian communication styles often value the control of thoughts or emotions, Asian American women patients may be reluctant to disclose personal information and feelings to a health care provider. In addition, they may also be reluctant because they are unsure of how their privacy and confidentiality is being protected. This difference may produce uncertainty about consent or compliance or may result in the medical needs or concerns of Asian American women patients to be overlooked.

NAWHO recognizes that there are three main levels of barriers to breast and cervical cancer outreach, education, and screening practices in Asian American communities: institutional, community, and provider level barriers. These barriers may affect women's ability to seek and receive screening. At a minimum, health care providers should be aware of these confounding conditions of life that Asian American women may experience and that can influence their knowledge and receipt of breast and cervical cancer screenings. In response, health care providers should consider these barriers when developing outreach or service programs to Asian American women.

Institutional Barriers

Institutional barriers are those which emerge from the dominant institutions or systems of society (i.e., the medical system, the predominant economic system, infrastructures, public perceptions, etc.) and which may be beyond the individual's immediate or perceived ability to overcome or change.

These can include:

The Socioeconomic Environment

The social and economic conditions of life for Asian American women may confound their knowledge of and access to health care, and to breast and cervical cancer screenings in particular. The effects of poverty such as: inadequate education, substandard and/or crowded housing, chronic malnutrition or other chronic health conditions, psychosocial stress, exposure to negative environmental agents, unemployment or underemployment may all be present in the socioeconomic environment of Asian American women and may impede their access to breast and cervical cancer screening services.

The Health Care System

Systems of health care service delivery may create barriers to accessing breast and cervical cancer screenings for all women, and for Asian American women in particular. Asian American women may face rising medical costs, have no insurance or be underinsured, or have inadequate or no government-sponsored health care. Because Asian American women may be in economically disadvantaged positions, high medical costs combined with lack of insurance can be a major deterrent to seeking care. In addition, the lack of targeted health education and outreach to Asian American women about breast and cervical cancers—especially in immigrant and/or non-English speaking communities—combined with a lack of language-appropriate education materials or inter-preters results in little community awareness or action regard-ing these diseases. Moreover, after Asian American women are diagnosed with cancer, locating and accessing support services (i.e., support groups, oncology counseling) that are culturally and linguistically appropriate is virtually impossi-ble. Many health care systems do not provide support to can-cer patients postdiagnosis and/or during treatment.

Infrastructure

As is the case for many underserved communities, Asian American women may face a lack of social or government sup-port services that facilitate their access to health care and to breast and cervical cancer screenings. Lack of available or affordable transportation, lack of available or affordable child care, or lack of convenient health care resources may prevent Asian American women from seeking services.

Research

Social service programs, infrastructure development, educa-tional programs, and service-delivery systems may all be influenced by the results of scientific data and research that identify priority health needs and trends. Data regarding the health status of Asian Americans are inadequate, and the myth that Asian Americans are a healthy population or model minority has perpetuated the argument that targeted outreach and education about breast and cervical cancers is not needed by this community. This misperception has also fueled a lack of screening referrals for Asian American women by the medi-cal community. Moreover, scientific literature does not address the underlying cultural and historical events that have profoundly shaped the lives of immigrants.

Community Barriers

Community barriers are those that emerge from the common values and belief systems of a population. These common values and belief systems are not inherently negative, but, if/ when they differ markedly from the values and beliefs on which breast and cervical cancer screening behaviors depend, they may become barriers to care. These common values and belief systems can act on both an individual and collective level and can include:

Philosophical Beliefs

The Asian philosophical values surrounding self-concept, the role of the family, and the role of women may create a mindset that minimizes the individual health needs of Asian American women. Asian American women may be socialized to view themselves within a larger context that defines them according to the group to which they belong, in particular, their family, and which further places them in a submissive, accommodating, and self-sacrificing role. They may, therefore, fail to access preventive health care services for themselves, particularly breast and cervical cancer screening services. They may also neglect their own health needs as they work to ensure the overall health of their families.

Health Attitudes

Traditional beliefs about health and illness may influence Asian American women's health-seeking behaviors. The belief that illness is a condition over which individuals have no control may prevent Asian American women from seeking health care in general. The lack of orientation to preventive medicine may further prevent Asian American women from seeking early detection screenings, with women often being unaware of the need for breast and cervical cancer screening and diagnoses or uninformed about what those entail. In addition, the tendency to seek medical care only in the presence of acute symptoms and pain opposes recommendations for early detection screening.

American Medical System

Lack of familiarity and trust of American health care systems and a reliance on traditional health practices may prevent Asian American women from seeking breast and cervical cancer screenings, which rely heavily on modern technologies and have an emphasis on prevention. Meanings and connotations of early detection terms such as cancer or mammogram can differ across cultures and communities. Misunderstandings of such health vocabulary and the lack of adequate language translation in medical settings may further dissuade Asian American women from seeking services related to these diseases.

Modesty

Prohibitive gender-based concerns may restrict Asian American women from seeking their own health care services or from seeking services that focus on private areas of the body. Many cultural beliefs about women's bodies prohibit Asian American women from discussing or thinking about reproductive organs such as breasts. They may feel too modest to receive examinations for breast or cervical cancers, or they may feel that such services are not necessary. They may also object to seeing male physicians for these services. The extent to which community barriers exist depends largely on acculturation level. The less an individual is acculturated to life in the United States and to the American medical system, the more likely it will be that the individual subscribes to the same beliefs, fears, and gender roles that serve as the community-level barriers to accessing care. Level of acculturation should be considered when providing services to Asian American women.

Provider Level Barriers

Provider level barriers are those which emerge from the culture of health care service-delivery including the knowledge and sensitivity of physicians, nurses, technicians, or social workers. These barriers can manifest during interactions between health care providers and their clients. These can include:

Provider Attitudes

The lack of institutionalized cultural competency training means that many providers may not have the knowledge or tools to deal effectively with Asian American women. They may not view clients as individuals with differing levels of needs, knowledge, and fears and, consequently, not exhibit respect for clients as individuals. Due to many other factors that are out of physicians' control, many providers may also use a compartmentalized approach to women's health care, focusing only on the problems with which clients present themselves or with acute medical problems rather than on overall wellness.

Communication Strategies

NAWHO also developed a set of guiding principles for culturally competent communication to help providers improve the level of service to Asian Americans.

Be Prepared

Because language is key to understanding the needs of Asian American women patients, the involvement of professional medically trained language interpreters may be critical to successful communication, especially for Asian American women with poor English proficiency. Translated health education materials on breast and cervical cancers, early detection, and other health issues can also be used to supplement information communicated during a screening visit.

Be Flexible

Each Asian American woman will respond differently to the breast and cervical cancer early detection screening environment. Often their needs and concerns will correspond to levels of acculturation and familiarity with American medical settings. Health care providers should gauge such levels of familiarity and adjust interactions accordingly, such as the decision to use language interpreters or medical terminology. Health care providers should be prepared with multiple communication approaches in order to tailor communications to patient needs.

Be a Partner

The communication styles of Asian American women can differ from the modes of expression expected in the American medical setting. Such expectations, when they conflict with a patient's preferred communication style, can result in perceived disrespect. Health care providers should nurture patient participation in communication by becoming aware of and honoring their communication styles.

The Need for Language Interpretation Services

Another important communication strategy is to increase the use of language interpretation services. The increasing diversity of the United States population has expanded the definition of language capacity in the health care setting. A single service area or patient population might now include a great variety of languages and dialects as well as levels of English proficiency and familiarity with English medical terms. To ensure effective communication with all potential patients, health care providers must develop a system for achieving language capacity in their health care settings. Because bilingual health care providers may be scarce depending on location and language needs, an effective and practical solution for achieving language capacity is the use of external language interpretation services.

Interpretation Service Models

Bilingual health care providers are best positioned to provide language interpretation during a patient encounter. However, few health care settings have access to the number of bilingual health care providers needed to meet potential language needs. In lieu of this option, several models for interpretation services have been developed:

Professional Interpreters

A professional language interpreter is an on-site staff person who provides medical language interpretation for health care providers. Often certified in language interpretation by a regional or national agency, on-site professional language interpreters have specific training in medical terminology as well as interpretation ethics and techniques. Their language abilities are also carefully screened. Such individuals may be full-time staff or hourly contractors and may be hired through certification agencies or language banks. Cost and availability of interpreters may pose challenges to this model.

Telephone Interpretation Services

A typical telephone interpretation service language line is a commercial on-demand service for registered health care providers or organizations that can pro
vide a language interpreter by telephone for a wide variety of language needs. Though such services offer certified interpreters, such individuals may not be trained in medical terminology. Moreover, the process for interpretation on a language line requires the use of telephone technology. At best, a speakerphone should be used in this model and the language line should be carefully screened before contracting.

Bilingual Support Staff

A bilingual support staff is an on-site staff person with known language proficiency who can provide on-call language interpretation for health care providers, but who is not trained or certified in language interpretation. Because such individuals are not professional language interpreters, their language proficiency and medical vocabulary cannot be guaranteed. It is possible that such individuals may serve primarily as language translators, with content sacrificed. Providing bilingual support staff with language interpretation training can help address these concerns. Faced with few options for language interpretation, some health care providers may use family members or friends as interpreters. Sometimes, nonmedical personnel known to be bilingual may also be used.

The Role of the Language Interpreter

The use of a language interpreter in the health care setting introduces a third party into the patient/provider relationship. However, the role of the language interpreter is to sustain the critically important patient/provider relationship through the facilitation of effective communication, using the least invasive methods possible. To do so, language interpreters primarily serve as a conduit for verbal communication between provider and patient, using the full range of linguistic resources to maintain fidelity of communication. When necessary to maintain effective communication, however, language interpreters may also serve as cultural brokers who facilitate cultural understanding between provider and patient. The extent to which language interpreters extend their roles into cultural brokering will depend on the potential for misunderstanding, which may ultimately undermine communication.[6] Regardless of their role, certified language interpreters adhere to a strict set of ethics including confidentiality, accuracy, neutrality, and respect for providers and patients.[7]

Outreach Strategies

There is no one way to achieve effective outreach to Asian American women. Every situation, location, and community is unique and may require different outreach strategies. Moreover, multiple approaches to culturally competent outreach may be needed before the best alternative is discovered. In the end, increased utilization of breast and cervical cancer early detection services and community empowerment through public education are the primary goals of culturally competent outreach.

General Steps of an Outreach Plan

Though outreach plans may vary depending on the priority population and the focus of the program, there are three general steps for developing any outreach plan.

Understanding the Message

Before an outreach program can bring its messages to the community, the goals of these messages must be fully understood. What does the outreach program hope to gain from this effort? What will be the impact of these efforts on the community? More specifically, what is the current level of awareness of these messages in the priority population? Are there models from which the current program can seek guidance?

Crafting the Message

Community responsiveness to a public education message relies on the appropriateness of the message, how that message is presented, and whether the messages reflect knowledge about the audience being targeted. Language, images, color, tone, and more can all affect the impression that a message makes on the community. This tailored approach can help optimize community receptivity to positive health behavior changes.

Moving the Message

A health promotion message is all but ineffective if the priority population never receives it. Thus, the final component of any outreach plan is a strategy to move the message into the priority population. It is the responsibility of health care providers and agencies to locate the most effective distribution and promotional vehicles. Where will Asian American women see a poster about breast and cervical cancers? What media do Asian American women read?

Five Essential Components of a Culturally Competent Outreach Plan

A successful, culturally competent outreach plan should include the following components.

Knowledge of the Community

Adequate knowledge of the community—including its beliefs and barriers, work and recreation patterns, health needs and concerns and more—is an essential component of an effective and culturally competent outreach plan.

Partnerships with the Community

To facilitate knowledge and dissemination of information and services to the community, effective community messengers and partner organizations must be identified, recruited, and trained. These partners should be included in the decision making and planning of outreach efforts, generating innovative and creative ways to promote health education and services, and increase responsiveness by the target audience.

Appropriately Tailored Messages

Messages should be crafted and produced in ways that are responsive to the priority population and to Asian American women in particular. These messages should be ethnic- (i.e., Asian ethnic subgroups), gender-, and age-specific and should incorporate the beliefs and values as well as address the needs and concerns of the priority population. Moreover, these messages should be presented in ways that are appropriate to the education-, literacy-, language-, and access-capabilities of the priority population.

Mobilized Networks and Media Plan

To effectively disseminate the messages of an outreach program, a system of networks in the community with access to the community must be mobilized. Community partners must be motivated, trained, and given the resources to act as spokespeople and share outreach messages with their constituents; appropriate Asian and ethnic media outlets must be identified, notified, and given the resources to publicize information and available services to the community. A critical component of any outreach program should be a clearly articulated media plan that could include developing a media database, press releases, or press packets.

Sustainable Service Systems

An outreach plan will facilitate a long-term positive health relationship with the community only if service delivery systems are appropriately designed to accommodate the community once outreach messages are received. Culturally competent service delivery programs for Asian American communities should similarly reflect the guidelines for outreach programs. They should strive for innovation and creativity based on a foundation of knowledge of the community. They should include internal policy or personnel improvements that facilitate increased utilization. Moreover, they should be given appropriate resources to sustain the momentum generated once the initial effort is complete.

Guiding Principles for Culturally Competent Outreach

Though outreach strategies may vary depending on the priority population and the focus of the program, there are four general principles for developing any outreach plan.

At Every Level, Involve the Community

Attempts to reach a community without knowing the community are often inappropriately designed and poorly received. This is especially true with the Asian and Pacific Islander community that represents more than fifty different ethnic backgrounds, each with varying belief systems and barriers, among other situational, historical, social, and economic differences. An effective outreach program will need to consider these characteristics unique to each Asian American community and tailor its design accordingly, incorporating community participation in all phases of the program.

In Every Encounter, Use Community Partners

Outreach programs that attempt to reach communities as diverse and varied as the Asian American community can face obstacles such as not having sufficient knowledge, experience, or access to reaching and serving Asian American women. A culturally competent approach to outreach must include innovative and creative community partnerships to educate and serve the community. Effective partners can be organizations, community leaders, or Asian media outlets— virtually any avenue through which Asian American women can be reached and served.

With Every Message, Educate Whole Families

Cultural and social beliefs about gender may restrict many Asian American women from taking charge of their own health care. They may defer their own health care for that of other family members or resist seeking screening services out of fear that a cancer diagnosis may bring shame on their families. Due to these diverse pressures, educating women in isolation from their families may deter long-term health-seeking behaviors. Accurate messages must be targeted to whole families and communities as well to facilitate an environment in which Asian American women can seek early detection without barriers or fears. Outreach messages and strategies should not ignore the context of Asian American women's lives.

As a Guiding Perspective, Look to the Long Term

Just as it takes time for providers to know communities, so too does it take time for communities to know providers. Outreach programs targeted to Asian American communities should incorporate a long-term perspective, with a willingness to invest time and resources in developing a positive health relationship with communities over time.

Training The Trainers

The *Communicating Across Boundaries* training has been successfully developed and implemented by NAWHO and program partners across the country for more than five years, 1997 through 2002, and has been met with widespread praise and consistently positive results. To date, more than 850 health care providers in eight states have been trained at a NAWHO training, conducted in a variety of locations, including rural and urban sites, sites on the West coast and East coast and in the Midwest, and sites with established as well as emerging Asian American populations.

Today, the *Communicating Across Boundaries* training is poised for implementation in additional new sites and for additional new provider and Asian American communities across the country. The project evolved in 1999 with the addition of a cultural competency training curriculum and Trainers' Institute to give health care providers the knowledge and skills they need to reach Asian American women for screening to reverse life-threatening trends. By "training the trainers," NAWHO is now able to increase the program's influence exponentially while also nurturing and building partnerships with state-sponsored cancer control programs, national cancer agencies, and local and regional community-based organizations to effectively organize on the widest possible scale for the survival of Asian American women.

CHAPTER EIGHT

Transforming Information Into Action

The National Asian American Diabetes Education Campaign

Imagine an elderly Chinese woman telling her doctor in broken English that she's not feeling well. After a series of tests, the doctor makes his diagnosis: diabetes. To help him talk to her about the disease, he enlists the help of her son. However, the son grew up in the United States and speaks little Chinese, so many of the doctor's instructions get lost in the translation.

Another woman talks of coming to America: "The land of opportunity provided me with almost everything, including a variety of tasty foods. After enjoying all the delicious foods, I forgot that I probably had too much of everything."

She went to her doctor, was diagnosed with diabetes and prescribed medication, so, she thought she was cured. Two years later, she went for another checkup and was shocked to find out that she still had diabetes.

"I was very scared and depressed when I found out this horrible news," she told an interpreter. Soon she was on dialysis three times a week, and, after six years on dialysis, she had to have one kidney removed.

"Having this condition made my life very miserable. I don't have a clear understanding of why I have diabetes and what caused it because I don't understand English. Sometimes when I go to the doctor, my children interpret for me. But their English is limited, and I am sure some explanations are lost in the translation. Some people have told me not to eat too many sweets, but some people have told me to have some candies ready just in case I get tired and sweaty. It is very confusing. As I understand it, I have to eat a little at a time. The doctor told me to exercise, but I never do because I get tired too quickly."

These stories illustrate the great need for simple, culturally appropriate diabetes education for the estimated 750,000 Asian Americans who have diabetes, many of which have limited English language skills. Thousands more have little awareness of their risk for the disease.[1]

In addition to language differences, other barriers to diabetes care for Asian Americans include lack of health insurance, scarcity of culturally and linguistically competent health care providers, and low utilization of preventive health care. These obstacles put Asian Americans at great risk for serious complications including blindness, kidney failure, amputation, and heart disease. Diabetes is the fifth leading cause of death for Asian Americans between the ages of forty-five and sixty-four, but with self-management that combines changes in diet, exercise and medication, diabetics can lead fulfilling lives.[2]

Diabetes is a serious health problem for all Americans. Researchers estimate that 15.7 million people or 5.9 percent of the United States population suffers from this chronic, incurable disease. However, only 10.3 million cases of diabetes have been diagnosed, leaving an estimated 5.4 million people unaware of their risks.[3]

While most Asian Americans know a friend or relative who has diabetes, the disproportionate burden of the disease on Asian Americans is rarely discussed, leading Asian Americans to feel that they are not at risk. In fact, Asian Americans are at an even greater risk for diabetes than Caucasian men and women. According to the National Health Interview Survey, Type 2 diabetes, the most common form of diabetes that typically strikes after age forty, occurs in 2.4 percent of Asian American women and 3.4 percent of Asian American men, compared to 2.4 percent of Caucasian women and 2.5 percent of Caucasian men.[4]

Extensive local research shows an even higher prevalence for diabetes among some Asian groups. One study in Washington state of second-generation Japanese Americans between the ages of forty-four and seventy-four revealed diabetes rates of 20 percent in men and 16 percent in women.[5] Another study of elderly Chinese Americans in Boston showed rates of 12.5 percent in men and 13.3 percent in women.[6] And studies in Hawaii have shown that Asian Americans have prevalence rates at least twice as high as Caucasians living there.[7]

And although the rates of diabetes are similar in men and women, diabetes tends to be more severe in women, putting them at higher risk for heart disease, stroke, cardiac failure, blindness, and diabetic coma.[8]

Asian American children are also increasingly at risk for diabetes due in large part to obesity and lack of physical activity. Diabetes can occur in two forms—Type 1 and Type 2. In Type 1 diabetes, which typically develops in children and young adults, the body destroys cells that make insulin. Asian Americans are at a lower risk for

Type 1 diabetes. In Type 2 diabetes, the pancreas makes insulin, but the body is unable to properly use it. Until recently Type 2 diabetes was largely an adult's disease. However, it's now estimated that as high as 45 percent of newly diagnosed children have Type 2 diabetes.[9]

While Type 1 diabetes cannot be prevented, there is strong evidence that the risk for Type 2 diabetes can be reduced with lifestyle changes including a proper diet and regular exercise. For this reason, the American Diabetes Association recommends that overweight Asian American children be tested biannually for the disease starting at age ten.

Diabetes is a disease that must be managed carefully, so Asian Americans who either don't know they have diabetes or don't understand what they need to do to manage it are in critical need of information.

In 1999, NAWHO made education on diabetes management an urgent priority. From 1999 through 2001, NAWHO reached out to more than four hundred diabetes educators and practitioners in four cities nationwide with "Making a Difference: A Symposium for Action on Asian Americans and Diabetes.

In 2002, NAWHO extended its efforts with *Transforming Information Into Action: The National Asian American Diabetes Education Campaign*. By joining forces with the CDC and the National Diabetes Education Program (NDEP), NAWHO awarded $175,000 in grants to five community-based organizations to increase diabetes knowledge, screenings, and utilization of care services among Asian Americans and to improve cultural competency among the health care providers who serve them. NAWHO partnered with groups in New York, Georgia, Oregon, Illinois, and Hawaii and provided innovative outreach education such as cooking demonstrations led by certified nutritionists, stress management and diabetes seminars, nutrition and meal plans, and group exercise classes.

These programs also helped Asian Americans understand the risk factors for diabetes and promoted proper screening for early diagnosis.

Risk Factors for Asian Americans

- ◆ Obesity
- ◆ Family history of diabetes
- ◆ Delivery of a baby weighing more than nine pounds or previous diagnosis of gestational diabetes, which develops or is first noticed during pregnancy

Diabetes is diagnosed through blood tests that measure the levels of glucose (sugar) in the blood. However, Asian Americans face numerous challenges that make access to these basic screenings difficult and costly. More than 15 percent of Asian American and Pacific Islander women and 17 percent of men lack health insurance, which is a significant factor in promoting the use of preventive health care.[10] Uninsured rates vary widely across Asian American populations.

A 2001 study from The Commonwealth Fund found that one in five Asian American adults between the ages of eighteen and sixty-four is uninsured or has been uninsured at some point in the past year, with especially high rates for Korean and Vietnamese Americans. Asian Americans are also less likely than the overall population to seek preventive health care services. Only 41 percent of Asian Americans report having had a physical exam in the past year, and 70 percent having had their blood pressure checked, compared to 48 percent and 79 percent for the overall population.[11]

These education efforts reached more than four thousand Asian Americans in 2002 alone with culturally and linguistically appropriate information and educational materials about diabetes to promote early screening and healthy lifestyles. NAWHO has also launched a media campaign targeting more than two hundred Asian and non-Asian media venues with radio and print public service announcements translated into eleven Asian languages. These messages involve Asians living with diabetes in outreach efforts to "put a face" on the disease that is familiar, making Asians realize that they are at risk. These individuals share their experiences to reduce the stigma surrounding diabetes and show other Asian Americans how they can successfully manage the disease.

Mr. Wong, a retired butcher from Oakland, California, is one of these individuals who has been willing to tell his story to help others. Mr. Wong says that when he found out that he had Type 2 diabetes, it was initially hard for him to accept the fact.

But unlike many Asian Americans who do little to manage the disease, Mr. Wong transformed the information he was being given about diabetes into action. He says he told himself, "I am going to beat this thing!"

Following his doctor's advice, Mr. Wong enrolled in diabetes education classes at the Summit Diabetes Center in Oakland. There he learned how to manage his diabetes by changing his diet and getting regular exercise. He replaced hamburgers and steaks with vegetables and moderate portions of lean meat. He also started walking regularly.

"You don't have to change your whole life," Mr. Wong says. "You just have to pay more attention to your health and make sure your life is balanced.

Mr. Wong is living proof that information can save lives. By allowing us write about his personal story in a NAWHO newsletter, Mr. Wong is reaching out to many other Asian

Americans with diabetes with the important message that they can lead productive lives.[12]

Self-management of diabetes typically involves a combination of nutrition, physical activity, and medication. The traditional Asian diet tends to be well balanced, relatively low in fat, relies upon less processed food, and doesn't promote snacking or dessert. However, the incorporation of American foods and eating habits—which include many foods that are high in fats and sugar, as well as highly processed foods and unhealthy snacks—has proven problematic for some Asian Americans, especially those with diabetes. Some studies have shown that Asian Americans who stick to a more traditional Asian diet have a lower prevalence of diabetes and that those who consume a primarily American diet had the highest prevalence of diabetes.[13]

Eating healthy to help reduce the risk for or manage diabetes involves preparing foods with less oil and salt, and choosing more vegetables and other high-fiber foods. Steaming and boiling are healthier cooking methods than deep-frying. Polyunsaturated oils and low-sodium seasoning are recommended over butter and lard. Cutting down on sugary soft drinks and sweets also helps.

Healthy Foods

Tofu
Soybeans
Green, leafy vegetables, such as:
    bok choy, mustard greens, kale
Fish
Chicken without the skin
Lean meats in moderate portions
Low-fat or non-fat milk

Foods to Avoid

Deep-fried foods
Butter, lard or heavy cream
Sugary snacks or sodas in large amounts
High-salt dishes
Red meat in large portions

Keeping active is also an effective self-management strategy. However, studies have shown that 57 percent of Asian American/Pacific Islander men and 65 percent of women lead sedentary lives.[14]

A contributing factor to this inactivity is the traditional belief among many Asian American cultures that being overweight means prosperity and is a blessing. Also in many Asian languages, the word exercise carries negative connotations.

These education materials explain that by keeping active, Asian Americans can lower their blood pressure and cholesterol levels, achieve healthy body weights, relieve stress, and increase their bodies' sensitivity to insulin, which is the primary medication used in diabetes treatment. The materials promote physical activities that can be incorporated easily into daily life such as walking, gardening, and housework, as well as yoga, tai chi, dancing, and stretching.

The proper use of diabetes medications can be difficult for Asian Americans who do not receive the proper information from their health care providers. The most common diabetes drugs are oral medications and injectable insulin. However, these medications are expensive, and to save money, many Asian Americans are using medications improperly, without realizing the risk they are taking.

Robin Chin, a pharmacist with CVS Corporation, says that in her many years as a pharmacist, she has seen Asian Americans take their prescribed medication only when they feel hyperglycemic, or stretch the medication, taking only small portions of the prescribed dosage to make it last longer. Another essential component of diabetes self-management is careful monitoring of blood sugar levels. But Robin has also seen many Asian Americans ignore directions for proper usage of test strips.

"Some people cut test strips in half and wash the strips for re-use," Robin says. "On the other end of the spectrum are the people who believe that if one pill is good, then two must be better."

By helping health care professionals provide culturally competent education and reaching the diverse Asian American community with information about reducing risk, screening and self-management in their own languages, NAWHO's *Transforming Information Into Action* campaign is working to prevent this type of dangerous behavior. Although the work must continue, we are reaching more people today with important health care information than ever before.

In 2002, NAWHO joined with the NDEP and the American Diabetes Association to urge Asian Americans with diabetes to carefully manage their blood pressure and cholesterol along with their blood sugar following new studies that show a strong link between diabetes and heart disease. Central to this effort is NAWHO's new diabetes web site portal at www.nawho.org that provides fact sheets and patient information materials in English, Cambodian, Chinese, Hmong, Korean, Tagalog, Thai, and Vietnamese languages. The portal campaign entitled *Take Care of Your Heart* also provides interactive features such as discussion boards, scheduled chats, polls, and a calendar of events to promote collaboration, feedback, and discussion to help reduce the risk for the life-threatening consequences of diabetes and reduce the disparity of diabetes among Asian Americans.

CHAPTER NINE

Sharing Responsibility

Exploring the Role of Asian American Men in Reproductive Health

In many Asian cultures, special significance is placed on the male children in a family—particularly the first male child. For centuries, the arrival of a baby boy has been a time for great celebration. While this preference certainly brings with it special privileges, it also carries intense responsibility. The male child is looked upon to carry on the family lineage, provide support for the family, and care for parents in their old age. The bias certainly is waning, but the ghost of ancestral ways continues to color thoughts and behaviors creating great disparities and health risks for the Asian American community.

Since NAWHO began its work in the Asian American community in 1993, the reproductive health needs of Asian American women have been a priority. In the Asian American community—just as in the whole of American society—reproductive and sexual health issues are at the forefront of the discussion and promotion of gender equality. Since its inception, NAWHO has worked to address the reproductive health needs of Asian American women and families using numerous strategies in research, education, and public policy. As a result, we have increased the body of knowledge about Asian women's reproductive health status and taken this information to the masses, educating health care providers, the Asian American community, and the general population to dispel myths and stereotypes that hurt this grossly underserved group of women. These efforts have also enabled us to provide recommendations to policymakers and opinion leaders for improving reproductive health policies for Asian Americans as well as to advocate for the continuance of individual freedoms to fully exercise reproductive and sexual health decisions.

While NAWHO was building the advocacy base to promote the health of Asian American women, we realized that the absence of knowledge about the reproductive health practices and behaviors of men had a profound effect on our efforts. To further our work, it was apparent that we needed to increase our knowledge about the reproductive health of Asian American men. In their dominant role in traditional Asian culture as well as their roles as partners, parents, and consumers, men heavily influence community views of health issues, the consequent utilization of health care services, and the extent to which Asian American women value their own reproductive health and wellness.

So, in 1999, with support from the Richard and Rhoda Goldman Fund, The Moriah Fund, the Open Society Institute and the Public Welfare Foundation, NAWHO began the first national study on reproductive and sexual health of Asian American men.

This groundbreaking study, called *Sharing Responsibility*, took the body of knowledge that NAWHO had amassed a step further by filling this critical gap in knowledge. The study's ultimate goal was to enable Asian American women and men to make more informed decisions about their own reproductive and sexual health.

In 1995, NAWHO's earliest study, *Perceptions of Risk,* had examined the various factors that were keeping Asian American women from accessing reproductive health services. Through interviews and focus groups with Asian American women of different ethnic, generational, and socioeconomic backgrounds, as well as their health care providers, *Perceptions of Risk* found that Asian American women felt that their risk was low, and so they didn't access preventive health care. Cultural norms, including silence and shame surrounding health issues—particularly sexual health and menstruation—as well as relationship dynamics and a lack of access to information about sexual and reproductive health were the primary factors associated with the perception of low risk.

In this survey, one service provider recalled an older woman who had vaginal bleeding for more than ten years without seeking attention. The woman eventually told the practitioner that she had felt too embarrassed to seek help and that if she had been able to endure the problem in the past, she should continue to endure it. The woman was eventually diagnosed with cancer.

Another health practitioner told us about a woman who had a positive chlamydia test but refused to believe the results. The practitioner explained to the woman that chlamydia was a sexually transmitted disease (STD), but the woman kept saying that she was a faithful wife so the test couldn't have been accurate. The test was repeated with the same results, but the woman wanted a third test. Finally she came in for treatment, but didn't bring her husband.

Perceptions of Risk further found that many Asian American women didn't know the difference between private hospitals, insurance hospitals, county hospitals, and community clinics, so they could not make informed choices about the kinds of services they could afford or receive.

In 1997, NAWHO conducted a California statewide contraceptive technologies survey that showed that the majority of Asian American women were sexually active: 67.4 percent of the sample reported having at least one sexual partner, with the average number of sexual partners for those who were sexually active being 4.0, and the average age of first sexual intercourse being 18.5 years old. The survey, which was titled *Expanding Options*, showed almost 50 percent of the 674 Asian American women surveyed had not visited a health care provider within the last year for reproductive or sexual health services, and 25 percent had never visited one in their lives.

Furthermore, Asian American women were not adequately protecting themselves against pregnancy. For example, 61 percent of the sexually active women stated that they did not always use contraceptive methods during sex. The top reason given by 28.5 percent of the sample for not always using contraception was "monogamy/trust of partner." The next most common answers were "didn't have it during sex" (16.6 percent) and "partner doesn't want to use any" (11.5 percent).

From this information alone, we knew that Asian American women were sexually active but were not being educated about their sexual and reproductive health, resulting in great risk for unwanted pregnancy as well as cervical cancers, STDs, and HIV. Our hope was that by studying Asian American men, *Sharing Responsibility* would provide us with the information needed to develop broad-based, comprehensive strategies that would enable us to achieve higher levels of public health in the Asian American community as a whole.

During this time, the HIV/AIDS epidemic had prompted increased attention by the public health community of researchers, policymakers, and service providers to the roles that men play in sexual relationships and their impact on healthy behaviors. The need for communication about infection and protection, as well as the need for treatment of all sexual partners to reduce the spread of HIV and other STDs was making it necessary to address men in the entire context of their relationships—as providers, partners, and parents—rather than simply distributing contraceptive devices in hope that they would be used.[1]

While researchers had begun to explore the roles of men in sexual and reproductive health, before NAWHO's *Sharing Responsibility* study, no comprehensive national survey had been conducted on the reproductive and sexual health behaviors of Asian American men. There had been a number of local research initiatives focusing on specific segments of the Asian American community.

Many of these previous studies had determined that while there is a perception that Asian American communities are at relatively low risk of contracting HIV, in reality, the risk in some communities was considerable and growing. One study of students found that Asians were less likely to have heard of AIDS than students from other ethnic groups, while at the same time, HIV rates within Asian American communities were increasing.[2]

Sharing Responsibility significantly raised awareness about men's behaviors and choices and the important relationship of these actions to the health of their partners. The survey was conducted from March 17 through May 2, 1999, with 802 Asian American men between the ages of eighteen and sixty-five in the consolidated metropolitan statistical areas of California and New York states. The men were asked questions regarding their knowledge, attitudes, and behaviors regarding reproductive and sexual health issues. Data collection and cross-tabulations were conducted by Survey Methods Group at its Computer Assisted Telephone Interviewing facility in San Francisco. The response rate was 58 percent in California and 46 percent in New York. Most of the men surveyed (71.1 percent) were between the ages of eighteen and thirty-four, and considered to be in their peak reproductive years. More than half of them (53.6 percent) were single. Further, 75.1 percent of the respondents were not born in the United States. More than half of the men (59.4 percent) were Chinese American, 12.0 percent were Korean American, and 22.4 percent were Vietnamese American.

Only 13.5 percent of men surveyed had no health care coverage at all, and 29.3 percent reported an income level between $25,000 and $50,000.

The survey results covered behaviors, attitudes, and knowledge. Its major limitation was that it was conducted in English, so was not reflective of the entire Asian American community.

Behaviors

Asian American men are as sexually active as the general US population of men.

- ♦ 86.6 percent of respondents reported having at least one sexual partner in the past year compared to 84 percent of US men who reported having had sex within the previous year in a 1998 Kaiser Family Foundation study.

Asian American men are not utilizing reproductive health services.

♦ Despite the low percentage of men without health care coverage, a vast majority of respondents (89.2 percent) had never seen a health care provider for reproductive health services such as family planning or sexually transmitted diseases. Less than half of the men surveyed (48.3 percent) reported that health care providers are a source for their health information.

Influenced by their perception of low risk, Asian American men are not always practicing safer sex.

♦ 82.9 percent of respondents felt they were not at risk for HIV, and 80.2 percent of Asian American men felt they were not at risk for any STDs.

♦ 60.3 percent of Asian American men surveyed had never been tested for HIV. Among respondents with $24,000 or less in annual household income, 71.3 percent had never been tested as compared to 52.1 percent with incomes in the $50,000 to $100,000 range.

♦ Almost half of the sexually active respondents (49.1 percent) were not always protecting themselves against STDs and unplanned pregnancies.

♦ Of the Asian American men who said they used condoms, only 31.5 percent said they always used this method of protection when engaging in sexual activity. The top reason for not using any type of protection was being in a monogamous relationship (29.6 percent).

♦ 63.4 percent of respondents who used protection said they were using it for the primary reason of preventing pregnancy, but only 8.0 percent of respondents were using it primarily to prevent STDs, and only 6.1 percent to prevent HIV infection.

♦ 26.3 percent of respondents who did not always use protection during sex had an unplanned pregnancy.

Attitudes

Asian American men feel responsible for reproductive health decisions.

♦ 81.9 percent of Asian American men surveyed said they fell a shared responsibility for making family planning decisions.

♦ 74.6 percent of respondents agreed that if a couple has never discussed birth control or condoms, the man should bring it up before having sex for the first time.

Asian American men support public funding for reproductive health services.

♦ The majority of men surveyed (79.1 percent) thought that legislators should support public health funding for family planning. Vietnamese men gave the highest rate of support—82.2 percent.

A majority of Asian American men are pro-choice.

♦ 76.8 percent of Asian American men surveyed supported a woman's choice to have an abortion.

♦ 40.9 percent of respondents said they would support a woman's decision in all cases and 35.9 percent only in certain cases.

♦ Respondents born in the United Stated and those who had lived for ten years or more in the United States were more likely to support a woman's decision to have an abortion than those who had been in the United States for less than ten years.

Knowledge

Asian American men look to the mass media for reproductive health information.

◆ Of men surveyed, the majority said they received their information from media and written sources. More than half reported relying upon health brochures (55.6 percent), while 68.3 percent reported getting their information from books, 68.3 percent magazines, and 65.1 percent television.

Condoms were by far the most recognized and most used birth control method among Asian American men.

◆ Vietnamese men surveyed were less likely to have heard of other birth control methods or behaviors than Chinese or Korean American men.

Various types of STDs were not widely recognized among Asian American men.

◆ Vietnamese men respondents were less likely to have heard of various STDs compared to Chinese or Korean American men.

◆ Asian American men who had been in the United States less than ten years were less likely to have heard of HIV/AIDS.

Overall, NAWHO's *Sharing Responsibility* study found that Asian American men and their partners were at a high risk for STDs and HIV since the majority of men surveyed were sexually active, did not always practice safer sex, and were not fully knowledgeable about STDs. This set of facts has an immediate impact on the health of their partners, placing them at tremendous risk for STDs and unplanned pregnancy. Though most of those surveyed had health insurance, they were not accessing reproductive health care, a critical gap not only because of the lack of utilization of testing for STDs and HIV but also because this was a missed opportunity for reliable health care information.

There are more than 11,500 new cases of reportable STDs occur among Asian Americans and Pacific Islanders each year.[3] The behaviors also may help to explain why Vietnamese women have the highest rates of cervical cancer of all racial and ethnic groups[4] since the STD Human Papillomavirus (HPV) is closely linked to cervical cancer.[5]

There is much work to be done to increase public health education and raise awareness with Asian Americans about their sexual and reproductive health, particularly their risk for STDs and HIV infection. The important opportunity identified by *Sharing Responsibility* is that Asian American men expressed a desire to be responsible decision-makers in sexual relationships. Respondents indicated strong feelings about shared responsibility for making family planning decisions as well as making decisions about using protection. Unfortunately their extremely low sense of personal risk for STDs and HIV infection had a much greater influence on their behavior.

Absent the feeling that they were at risk, feeling responsible for reproductive health matters just didn't translate into practice since only 50.9 percent of Asian American men surveyed said they always used protection, and then mostly to prevent pregnancy.

The age-old customs of Asian cultures are at work here, influencing Asian American men to express these feelings of responsibility that have been bestowed upon males for centuries. For this reason, education conducted in the context of being responsible to partners and families has great potential to influence Asian American men. In addition to working to increase the understanding of risk, public health programs must also educate health care providers to understand the needs of this population and take every opportunity to encourage open communication about reproductive health matters with their Asian American male patients.

Therefore, open communication within the family will be the most powerful prevention tool in the area of reproductive health. A number of efforts will have to come together to influence positive change:

1. NAWHO has launched a Family Communications Campaign to get parents to take responsibility as educators within their families. If Asian American parents will provide their children with medically accurate sex education information at home, addressing these issues as early as possible—before daughters and sons become sexually active—it will certainly promote more responsible adult behavior.

2. Involving Asian men in our work is important so that they can translate their feelings of responsibility into action by utilizing family planning services, using condoms, and getting tested for infection and HIV.

3. Educating Asian women about getting regular Pap smears and gynecological exams is also important if they are to actively practice prevention. Many organizations, including the American Cancer Society, National Cancer Institute, American College of Obstetricians and Gynecologists, American Medical Association, American Academy of Family Physicians, and others recommend that Pap testing should begin annually at the onset of sexual activity or at age eighteen and continue less frequently at the discretion of the doctor and patient after three or more annual tests have been normal.

4. Also keeping older women aware that even though they are past menopause, they still need to have regular Pap tests to reduce their risks. Pap testing is necessary for all women except those who have undergone a hysterectomy in which the cervix was removed. Even in that case, Pap testing is necessary if the hysterectomy was performed because of cervical cancer or its precursors.[6]

Ultimately, good communication about reproductive health decisions between partners is the best prevention strategy. Risk cannot be reduced unless both partners practice safe behaviors. Men and women can lead the way by talking to their partners and their health care providers.

CHAPTER TEN

Silent Epidemic

Violence against Women in the Asian American Community

When I was a young girl living with my family in Seoul, I had a friend whose mother was a victim of abuse. One day my friend ran to our house crying that her dad was beating her mom. I grabbed her hand and ran with her back toward her house. A security guard was in the neighborhood, and I told him what was happening and that my friend and I needed his help. I remember that he was reading the newspaper, and he looked up and started laughing at us. Then he just went back to reading.

I felt so helpless. This situation seemed so obviously wrong, yet no one was going to do anything about it. This was the common attitude in Korea at the time. Women had little power in the family, and, if they were abused, they had no one to go to for help. Like my friend's mother, they kept quiet and endured the pain.

This is a snapshot of the type of domestic violence that occurs in many Asian countries. And since this treatment of women was legal, when these families immigrate to the

United States, it often continues. Even though there are laws in the United States protecting women from domestic violence, many Asian American immigrants don't understand their rights. And so the abuse continues—often into the next generation.

That is the second snapshot I want to give you—the one of violence against young Asian American women, who are also in danger. This snapshot is of a Korean American seventeen-year-old named Rene. Rene is the second of three children. Her parents came to the United States two months before she was born and brought their traditional Korean values with them. They moved in with her uncle's family.

Rene's parents are embarrassed by their poor English and never really learned to navigate American culture. The family's social and business circles are confined almost entirely to other Korean Americans. They distrust non-Asian medicine and social services—in large part because of all the bad experiences their friends and neighbors have had—and they're unaware of the kinds of care and assistance that are available.

Rene's father is a strict and often physical disciplinarian, just as his own father was. Growing up, Rene often saw her uncle slap her aunt. Violence is part of her home environment. It's part of her family culture.

When she was fourteen, her uncle sexually assaulted her. This was a different and terrifying kind of violence, and it deeply frightened her. Yet she couldn't tell anyone. Certainly not her parents. In their culture, such abuse does not create a victim—only shame. True to her upbringing, Rene kept silent rather than bring her shame upon the entire family and likely be beaten for it.

It was exactly what her uncle expected, of course. Which is why he knew he could get away with it.

At seventeen Rene was raped by one of her older brother's friends. This time her shame was compounded with fear—she was terrified that it would happen again. She withdrew from her family and friends and began cutting classes. She found excuses not to come home after school or on weekends until close to bedtime. Within weeks her B average in school plummeted. The sudden changes in her behavior raised her parents' suspicions that she was up to no good, which earned her more physical discipline.

Then something very fortunate happened. One of Rene's closest friends, a Vietnamese boy named Mike, became so alarmed at the changes he saw in her that even though he didn't know about the rape, he broke the silence. Mike was a student aide to one of the school's administrative secretaries, a non-Asian woman widely known as someone that students could talk to confidentially. Mike told her his concerns, and the secretary quickly agreed to do what she could.

The next day, Mike brought Rene to the secretary's office and convinced her that the woman could be trusted. Reluctantly, bit by bit, Rene began to talk. Not much at first. But gradually over the next several days, as her trust and confidence grew, she confided everything—about her family, about her uncle, and finally, in a torrent of tears, about the rape.

The secretary had taken intervention training and knew that Rene needed professional help. She also knew it was going to take time for Rene to reach the point where she would accept that help. For the time being, the secretary could do little but listen. But that seemed to be what Rene needed most. She stopped cutting classes. She began to hang out with her regular circle of friends again.

Then, less than a month after the rape, Rene missed her period. She knew what a pregnancy would mean to her family. Her parents would never believe that she'd been raped. And how she got pregnant wouldn't matter anyway. She would be beaten regardless of the circumstances. She would probably be sent away, and her family would be disgraced.

Rene felt trapped, and she knew of only one path of escape: she swallowed a bottle full of sleeping pills. Then she sat down and wrote her family a letter of apology for failing them. But as the pills began to take effect, she did something that just a couple weeks before never would have occurred to her. She telephoned the school and asked to speak with the secretary. The secretary had already left for the day, but the act of reaching out to someone triggered something in her, and she made a second phone call to her friend Mike.

There are thousands of young women like Rene. They are the real faces and real lives behind the grim statistics that point to a crisis of enormous proportions. Rene is one of the lucky ones. She survived to tell her story. The school secretary became her advocate, convincing not just her but her entire family to get professional counseling. And today Rene has a new life and great hopes for the future. The cycle of violence in her family is broken.

Violence against women happens in all types of intimate relationships and crosses economic, educational, cultural, racial, and religious lines. Nearly one-third of women murdered each year in the United States are killed by their current or former intimate partners. Approximately one million women are stalked each year, and one in thirty-six college women is a victim of an attempted or completed rape in each academic year. As a result, across the country, women live in constant fear that they will be attacked at home, at work, at school, or in public places.[1]

Violence against women is a worldwide health crisis. In recent years, the United States has made significant inroads

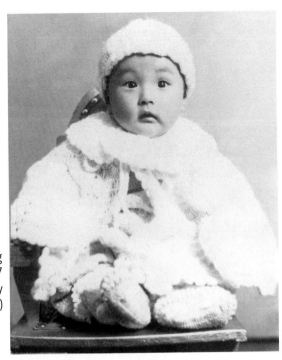

Mi Kyung Chung
November 23, 1967
(100 day
celebration)

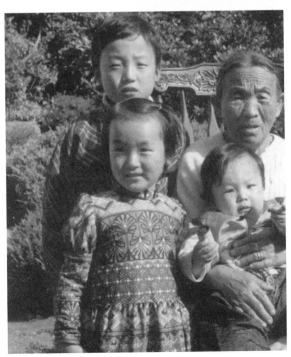

Kwangju, 1972
My older brother
Pil Ho (at 7),
Mi Kyung, five
years old, and
my grandmother
holding my baby
brother (one year
old). The right
side of the photo
has been cut off.
No longer in the
photo are my
older sister (she
was 8), standing
behind my
younger sister,
who was 3 years
old at the time.

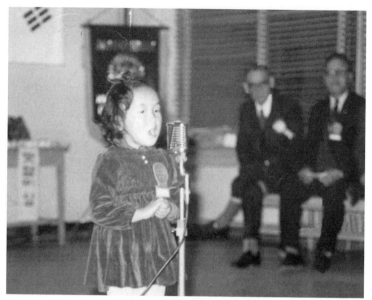

Mary at five years old

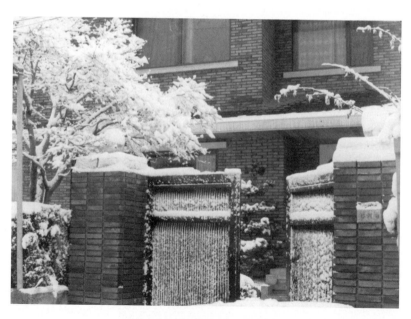

Our house in Seoul, 1978

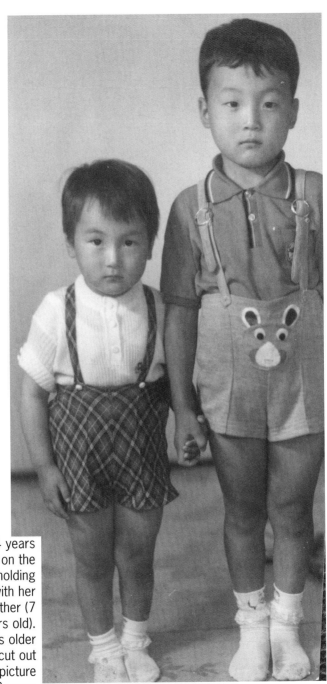

Mary (4 years old) is on the left, holding hands with her older brother (7 years old). Mary's older sister was cut out of the picture (she was 8 years old at the time).

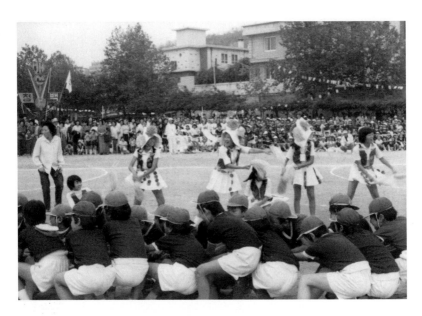

Seoul, 1979
I was a cheerleader in the sixth grade.

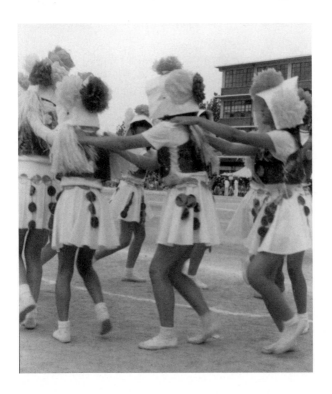

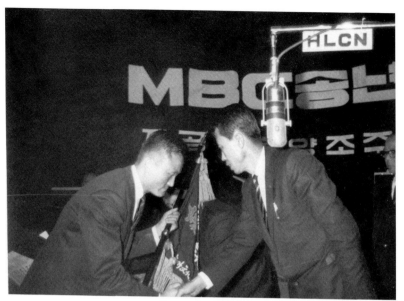

Kwangju, 1972
My dad (on the left). He regularly hosted the local
TV station's weekend program.

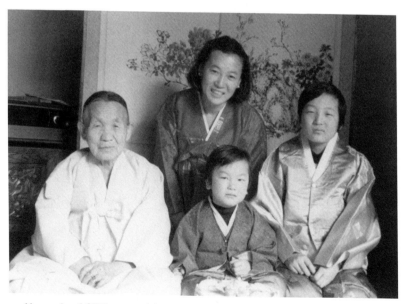

Kwangju, 1977—my older brother's eleventh birthday. My mother,
grandmother, and younger brother are also in the picture.

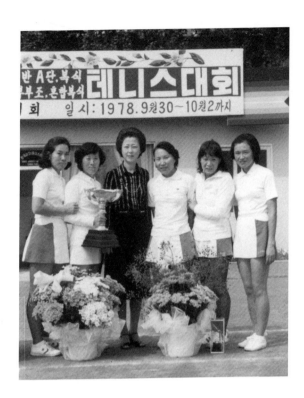

Kwangju, 1979
My mom
(2nd from right)
at a tennis
tournament

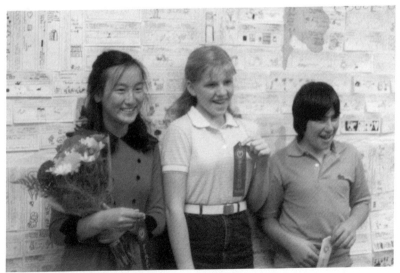

1981—Orange County Public Library Bookmark Contest.
Mary (on left) won first place.

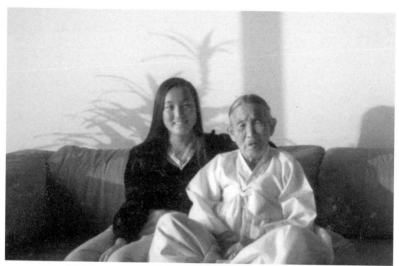

1982—Mary's grandmother visits Orange County
when Mary was in the eighth grade.

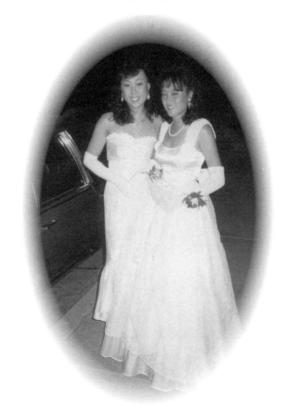

1986—Foothills
High School
Senior Prom.
Mary and friend
Patty

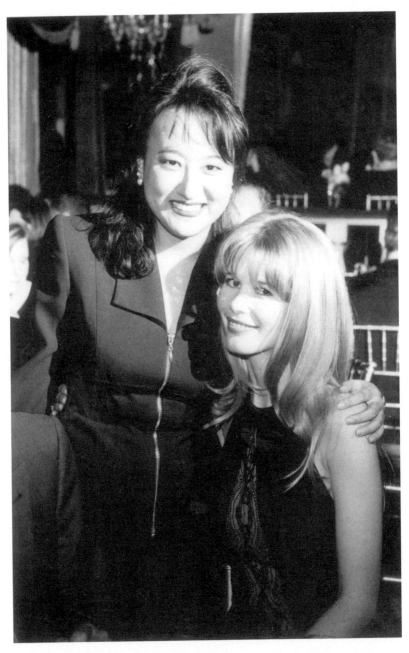

New York City, 1996—National Breast Cancer Coalition gala
Mary Chung, board member, with Claudia Schiffer

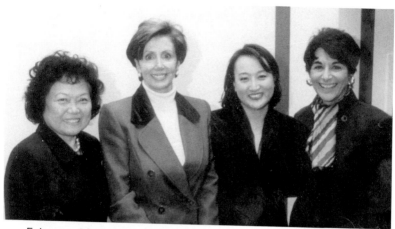

February 1998. Mary led more than 100 Asian American women community leaders from all over the country to Washington, DC for four days of intensive training on public policy and politics; one of the sessions focused on "congressional briefings by members on Asian American health issues."

Top (from the left): Congresswoman Patsy Mink, Congresswoman Nancy Pelosi, Mary Chung, Congresswoman Anna Eshoo.

Bottom: Attendees gather on the steps of the White House Old Executive Office Building

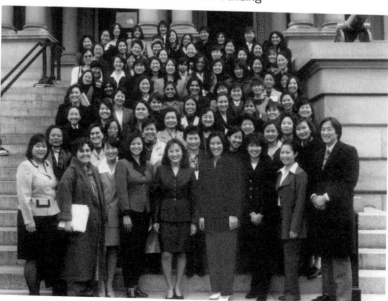

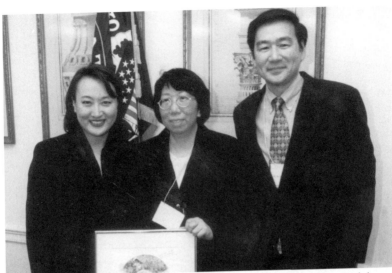

April 1999. During the second Asian American public policy training conference in Washington, DC, NAWHO honored Robin Chin, breast cancer survivor, for her advocacy work within the AA community. From the left: Mary Chung, Robin Chin, David Takeuchi, dean of sociology, graduate studies, University of Washington.

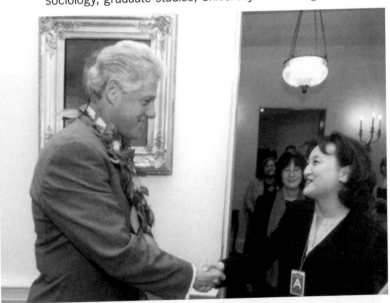

June 7, 1999—The White House. This was the signing ceremony when President Clinton signed an executive order creating the first White House Initiative on Asian Americans.

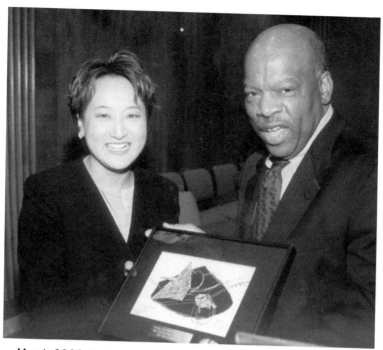

March 2000. During the third Asian American public policy training conference in Washington, DC, NAWHO honored Congressman John Lewis (above). Senator Dianne Feinstein (below) delivered the keynote speech on Asian Americans and politics.

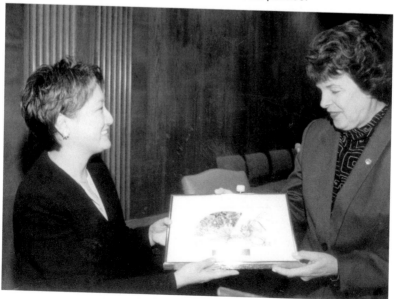

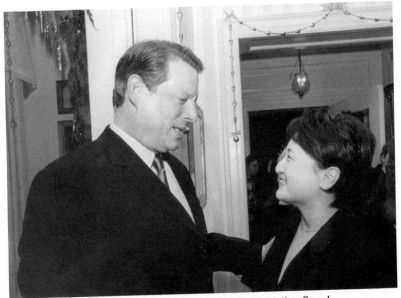

December 2000. A Christmas party at the Gore's,
following the presidential election.

Tipper Gore
invites you to a reception
in honor of
The National Asian Women's
Health Organization

on Tuesday,
the twenty-third of March
at ten-thirty o'clock
in the morning

The Vice President's Residence
34th Street and
Massachusetts Avenue, N.W.
Washington, D.C.

To Remind

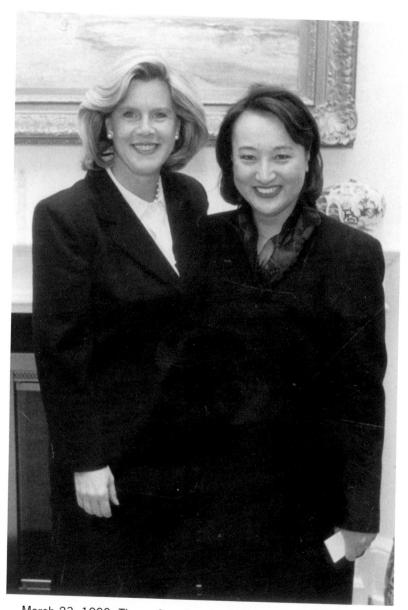

March 23, 1999. Tipper Gore honors Mary and the National Asian Women's Health Organization at the vice president's residence.

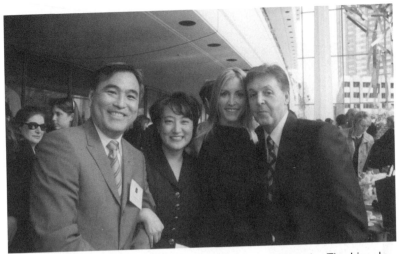

September 10, 2001—*RedBook Magazine* awards gala, The Lincoln Center, New York City. From the left: Dennis Hayashi, Mary Chung Hayashi, (honoree), Heather Mills McCartney (honoree), Paul McCartney.

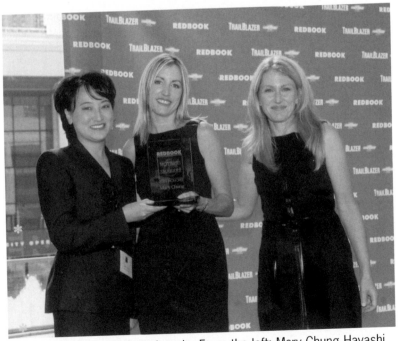

RedBook Magazine awards gala. From the left: Mary Chung Hayashi (honoree), Heather Mills McCartney (honoree), Jayne Jamison (vice president and publisher, *RedBook Magazine*).

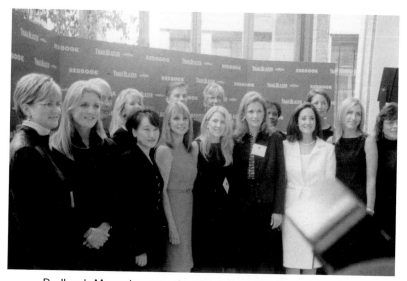

Redbook Magazine awards gala honorees, Sept. 10, 2001
The Lincoln Center

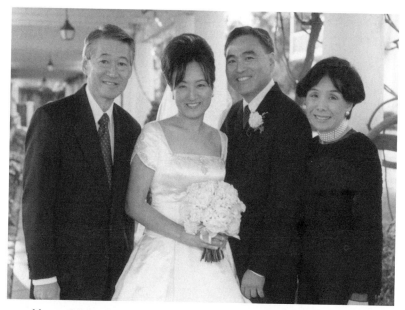

My wedding photo—October 6, 2001, Pasadena, Ritz Carlton.
From the left: Congressman Robert Matsui (officiated the ceremony),
Mary Chung, Dennis Hayashi, Doris Matsui

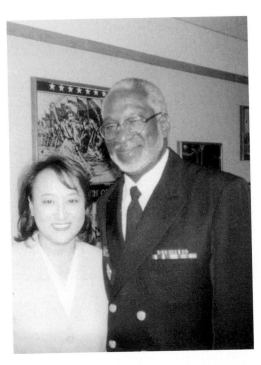

Top: Mary with former U.S. Surgeon General, Dr. David Satcher

Below, the first annual meeting of the Advisory Board of the Iris Alliance Fund on October 3, 2002 at the St. Regis Hotel in Los Angeles. Dr. Satcher, sitting next to Mary in the front row, center, is the honorary chairman of the Alliance Fund Board.

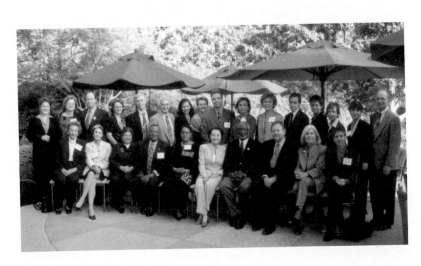

into prevention with efforts such as the Violence Against Women Act of 1994, which was strengthened 1998.

But even in communities where there are domestic violence shelters and rape crisis centers, many Asian American women are not seeking help. Traditional emphasis on saving face, which views talking about issues such as violence or rape as bringing shame upon the family, is keeping them silent. Also, as with my friend's mother in Seoul, Asian American immigrant women have been raised to honor and respect their husbands and totally depend upon them for support. They have few options for escape.

Many factors limit the ability of Asian American women to break free from the cycle of violence. Coming from a largely immigrant population with 61.4 percent being foreign-born, many Asian American women must face language barriers; lack of knowledge of legal rights under the Violence Against Women Act, including rights to public aid such as health benefits and financial assistance; issues surrounding their immigration status; lack of economic independence; and threat of retaliatory violence.

Given these circumstances and the fact that sexual violence had been found the most rapidly growing violent crime in America, in 2001 NAWHO began efforts to determine the impact of sexual violence, intimate partner violence, and stalking on Asian American communities.[2]

Many factors contributed to our decision to focus efforts on young women first. Violence prevention is a complex issue, particularly within the Asian American community, which is tremendously diverse in terms of language, culture, immigration status, and economic status. Since resources were limited, we had to determine where NAWHO could have the greatest impact by focusing on a particular population within the Asian community. Research by other institutions showed that college-age Asian American women were particularly at risk. Considering our core competency in Asian women, our National Leadership Network of young Asian women leaders, and a lack of resources to translate materials into many different languages, we decided to start with a population of college-age Asian American women that is primarily an English-speaking population.

When NAWHO began the effort, called *Silent Epidemic: A Survey of Violence Among Young Asian American Women*, existing data suggested that Asian American women were suffering from violence at rates comparable to or higher than the general population of women.

The National Violence Against Women (NVAW) Survey reported that 49.6 percent of Asian/Pacific Islander women had experienced physical assault, and 6.8 percent were victims of rape in their lifetimes compared to 51.9 percent and 17.6 percent for American women overall. Of these assaults, 25 percent were perpetrated by an intimate partner.[3] Overall, young women were found to be the most susceptible to acts of violence with 29.4 percent of female respondents to the NVAW Survey reporting that they experienced rape for the first time between the ages of eighteen and twenty-four.[4] Further studies had found that the highest rate of intimate partner violence was among women ages sixteen to twenty-four.[5]

But there was also evidence suggesting that the burden and degree of brutality of sexual violence and intimate partner violence against Asian American women was even greater. Local Massachusetts data showed that Asian Americans comprised 18 percent of the residents killed in 1997 as a result of violence in the home, though they represented only 3 percent of the state's population.[6]

The assumption was that reporting rates were skewed because of cultural norms that made Asian Americans less likely than other ethnic groups to perceive certain actions as abusive.[7]

The survey sought to fill the critical data gaps to best determine violence prevention strategies that would equip young Asian American women most at risk with the education and leadership skills needed to stay safe.

In April of 2001, NAWHO commissioned the Field Research Corporation to investigate the knowledge and awareness levels, incidence and prevalence, access to services, and education related to sexual violence and intimate partner violence among Asian American women. Because of the delicate nature of the topic, interviewers underwent intensive sensitivity training and made strict confidentiality agreements. In total, 336 women ages eighteen to thirty-four participated in the survey. Women represented the following ethnicities: 52 percent Chinese, 13 percent Korean, 12 percent Vietnamese, 11 percent Japanese, 4 percent Filipino, 2 percent Asian Indian and Thai, 2 percent other Asian, and less than 1 percent Hmong and Laotian. Potential participants were randomly selected from a list of phone numbers for individuals with Asian surnames in the Los Angeles and San Francisco metropolitan areas.

The survey was unique on several levels. Not only was it larger than previous studies, but also it was the first survey of its kind to examine various types of violence, including sexual violence, intimate partner violence and stalking, in the lives of Asian American women from California. The study did have its limitations. Even though it was larger than similar studies at the time, the sample size of 336 is not large enough to be representative of the entire Asian American community. Also, we assume, because of cultural factors, and under-reporting of violence data. Still, key findings do give us a greater understanding of the depth of attitudes and experiences among young Asian American women that confirmed they were at great risk.

Young Asian American women lacked knowledge about sexual violence and partner rape.

- ◆ A significant number of survey participants lacked understanding of the prevalence of acquaintance rape and rape by intimate partners. They had a limited scope of knowledge regarding the definition of rape, primarily viewing it as stranger rape. Although 94 percent of women surveyed agreed that rape is a serious problem, 19 percent did not believe that rape is most commonly committed by someone known by the victim, and 18 percent believed that rape does not happen between two people in a relationship.
- ◆ The findings underscored the need for acquaintance and date rape education and outreach programs.

The prevalence of violence was higher than previously reported.

- ◆ Young Asian American women faced various forms of violence at higher rates than previously estimated. 19 percent of the women said they had felt pressured to have sex without their consent since the age of eighteen. Of those who had felt pressured to have sex, 44 percent, which represents 8 percent of the total sample, had experienced completed rape. Of these completed rape victims, an intimate partner was the perpetrator 16 percent of the time.

Reports of physical violence and emotional abuse by intimate partners were also alarming.

- ◆ When survey participants were asked if an intimate partner had hurt or had attempted to hurt them by means of hitting, kicking, slapping, shoving, object throwing, or threatening their lives with a weapon, 12 percent answered, "yes." Because intimate partner violence includes both emotional and physical abuse, the survey also explored emotional abuse. When survey participants were asked if they had been repeatedly yelled at, sworn at, insulted, or had been a victim of excess jealousy and/or were denied access to family and friends, 26 percent said they had experienced at least one of these emotional abuses by an intimate partner.

♦ These results suggest that either emotional abuse is more common among Asian American women than physical abuse or that fewer stigmas exist with emotional abuse, resulting in increased reports from survey participants. The misperception that emotional abuse is "not really abuse" or that it is "more acceptable" perhaps enabled Asian Americans to talk about it more openly.

Existing stalking data was also misleading. One national study had reported that Asian/Pacific Islander women were "significantly less likely to be stalked" than the general population.[8] But Silent Epidemic produced far different results.

♦ When participants were asked if anyone had ever repeatedly followed or spied on them, had appeared at unexpected locations, had stood outside their home, school, or place of work, 14 percent said, yes." These results were higher than the national estimate of stalking for women overall of 8 percent.[9]

Access to sexual violence and intimate partner violence services were low despite the high incidence rate for victimization.

♦ Despite the high incidences of violence being reported by these young Asian American women, utilization of preventive care and treatment services was extremely low. Of those who identified themselves as college students, 95 percent said they had never used the student services on their campuses. When asked why, 23 percent said that they were not aware of them. The survey showed similar trends in usage of community services with 97 percent saying they had not used any of the social services available within their communities and 19 percent saying they did not know about them. With the prevalence rate as high as 18 percent, these statistics showed the great need for education and outreach.

This groundbreaking survey was a first step to understanding and addressing the realities of violence among young Asian American women. In disseminating the results, NAWHO is advocating that federal, regional, and local social service organizations prioritize Asian communities for inclusion in research, public education, and provision of services. Shortly after the *Silent Epidemic* survey was completed, NAWHO formed another partnership with the Division of Violence Prevention, National Center for Injury Prevention and Control, CDC. Called *Breaking the Silence: Culturally Competent Approaches to Violence Prevention for Asian American Women*, this evidence-based multitiered program addresses prevention strategies by working with young Asian American women who are at the greatest risk for sexual violence and intimate partner violence. Designed to train peer advocates, the program components include:

- ◆ A Prevention Conference and Leadership Institute to build leadership and advocacy skills of campus administrators and college students. Graduates of the program, returned to initiate activities at ten college campuses.
- ◆ A culturally competent educational curriculum to address barriers and stigmas that have been preventing Asian American women from speaking out and seeking help.
- ◆ NAWHO's Violence Prevention Site (www.nawho.org), which is an additional distribution channel for the latest

culturally responsible prevention information for the Asian American community.

As NAWHO continues to work on the violence-training curriculum, we are expanding strategic partnerships with colleges throughout California to hold additional conferences and trainings for campus administrators and young college-age Asian American women. Our hope is that these efforts will expand into model programs that will be replicated nationally.

CHAPTER ELEVEN

Keeping Hope Alive

America's Growing Mental Health Crisis

The statistics are staggering:

+ Each year, thirty thousand Americans will commit suicide— eighty-six a day.
+ Every day fifteen hundred people in the US will attempt to kill themselves.
+ For every two victims of homicide in this country, three people take their own lives.
+ In 1999, roughly one out of every thirteen US high school students reported making a suicide attempt in the previous twelve months.
+ Among adolescents and young adults in the United States, the rate of suicide has more than tripled since 1952, making suicide the third leading cause of death among fifteen- to twenty-four-year olds.
+ Even more disturbing, suicide is the sixth leading cause of death for five- to fourteen-year-olds.[1]

Words like "crisis" and "epidemic" are used sparingly in the public health arena, but when it comes to suicide, and the even larger problem of depression, which is a leading factor in most suicides, both words seem entirely appropriate as descriptors.

Women are at great risk to suffer from major depression at some point in their lifetime. According to *The Women's Health Data Book* published in 2001, about 13 percent of women will have a diagnosable depressive disorder in any given year, with one in five women experiencing an episode of major depression during her lifetime—twice the rate seen among men. *The Women's Health Data Book* goes on to explain that the average age of the first onset of major depression is in the mid twenties, with the peak occurring between twenty-five and forty-four.

The good news is that today more than ever before, mental health organizations such as the National Mental Health Organization, the Society for Women's Health Research and other advocacy groups are working with public officials to recognize mental health as an area that requires priority attention. Tipper Gore and her visible public advocacy work has been truly exceptional and has helped to raise awareness and reduce stigma.

In 1999, I was excited to be a participant in the first White House Conference on Mental Health and the first Secretarial Initiative on Mental Health from the Department of Health and Human Services. These groundbreaking activities set the stage for progress and focused attention on a problem that has long been swept under the rug. David Satcher, M.D., Ph.D., then surgeon general, brought the problems front and center and identified challenges for advocates, scientists, government officials, and consumers.

"Tragic and devastating disorders such as schizophrenia, depression and bipolar disorder, Alzheimer's disease, the mental and behavioral disorders suffered by children, and a range of other mental disorders affect nearly one in five Americans in any year, yet continue too frequently to be spoken of in whispers and shame," Satcher said. Adding that it was time that mental health flow into the mainstream of health.

Satcher went on to point out that while we do know more today about how to treat mental illness effectively and appropriately, even more than other areas of health and medicine, the mental health field is plagued by disparities in the availability of and access to its services.

"We have allowed stigma and a now unwarranted sense of hopelessness about the opportunities for recovery from mental illness to erect these barriers," Satcher said. "It is time to take them down."

In 1999, the US Congress had requested an Institute of Medicine study to assess the extent of disparities in the types and quality of health services received by US racial and ethnic minorities and nonminorities, which found that the biggest gap in health care for minorities was in mental health services.[2]

More recently this national tragedy was articulated by the President's New Freedom Commission on Mental Health, established in April 2002 by President George W. Bush as part of his commitment to eliminate inequality for Americans with disabilities. With mental illness being one of the leading causes of disability, the president directed the commission to identify policies that could be implemented by federal, state, and local governments to maximize the utility of existing resources, improve coordination of treatments and services, and promote successful community integration for adults with a serious mental illness and children with a serious emotional disturbance.

The New Freedom Commission noted that mental health was a serious public health challenge, was under-recognized as a public health burden, and that "one of the most distressing and preventable consequences of undiagnosed, untreated, or under-treated mental illnesses is suicide."[3]

While the general population suffers from mental illness at a rate of one in five, the Asian American community, particularly women, is experiencing even higher rates of mental illness. A NAWHO study of Asian American women published in 2001 reported that one of the first community studies of depression and Asian Americans conducted in the early 1970s found that 40 percent of Chinese Americans had a "sinking" depressed feeling.[4] Another study reported that 71 percent of Southeast Asians met the criteria for major affective disorder, a diagnosis that includes depression.[5] And in one survey of adolescents, 30 percent of Asian American girls reported depressive symptoms, compared to 23 percent of girls of other races.[6]

While the overall suicide rates for Filipino (3.5), Chinese (8.3), and Japanese (9.1) Americans are substantially lower than that for Caucasian Americans (12.8 per 100,000 per year), native Hawaiian youth have a higher risk of suicide than other adolescents in Hawaii. Also disturbing, older Asian American women have the highest suicide rate of all women over age sixty-five in the United States.[7]

When I first told the story of my sister's suicide at the NAWHO conference in 1995, I was overwhelmed by the number of people who came to me afterwards with their own stories about suicide. As I learned more about the problem, I realized how pervasive it is.

According to the Substance Abuse and Mental Health Services Administration, while overall prevalence rates of diagnosable mental illnesses among Asian American and

Pacific Islanders appear similar to those of the Caucasian population, when symptoms are scaled, Asian Americans show higher levels of depressive symptoms than do Caucasian Americans. Chinese Americans are more likely to exhibit somatic complaints of depression than are African Americans or Caucasians.

Additionally some Asian Americans experience syndromes tied to characteristics of their culture, such as *hwa-byung*, sometimes called suppressed anger syndrome. This syndrome is characterized by symptoms including constriction in the chest, palpitations, flushing, headache, dysphoria, anxiety, and poor concentration. Southeast Asian refugees in the United States are also at high risk for mental illness, specifically post-traumatic stress disorder (PTSD) associated with trauma experienced before and after immigration to America. One study found that 70 percent of Southeast Asian refugees receiving mental health care met the criteria to be diagnosed for PTSD. A study of Cambodian adolescents who survived concentration camps, found nearly half experienced PTSD and 41 percent suffered from depression a decade after leaving Cambodia.[8]

A 2001 report of the surgeon general, *Mental Health: Culture, Race and Ethnicity*, brought attention to disparities in access, quality, and availability of mental health services for racial and ethnic minority Americans.

The report, which was a supplement to the 1999 first-ever surgeon general's report on mental health, found that, although effective, well-documented treatments for mental illnesses are available, racial and ethnic minorities are less likely to receive quality care than the general population. Further it found that overall, only one in three Americans who need mental health services currently gets care. The critical result of the disparity, the report stated, is that minority communities bear a disproportionately high burden of disability from untreated or inadequately treated mental health problems and mental illnesses.

"While mental disorders may touch all Americans either directly or indirectly, all do not have equal access to treatment and services. The failure to address these inequities is being played out in human and economic terms across the nation—on our streets, in homeless shelters, public health institutions, prisons and jails," said Dr. David Satcher, who was the US surgeon general at the time. "The revolution in science that has led to effective treatments for mental illnesses needs to benefit every American of every race, ethnicity and culture. Everyone in need must have access to high-quality, effective and affordable mental health services. Critically, culture counts. That means we need to embrace the nation's diversity in the conduct of research, in the education and training of our mental health service providers and in the delivery of services."[9]

Asian Americans bear out this analysis with their extremely low utilization of mental health services when compared to other US populations. For example, one of the largest studies of Asian Americans to date, the Chinese American Psychiatric Epidemiological Study (CAPES) conducted in 1993 and 1994, examined rates of depression among more than 1,700 Chinese Americans in Los Angeles County and found that only 17 percent of those experiencing problems sought care. Among Asian Americans who use services, severity of disturbance tends to be high, perhaps because they tend to delay seeking treatment until symptoms reach a crisis point. Again shame and stigma are believed to figure prominently in the lower utilization rates as well as a lack of health insurance and lower utilization of Medicaid. According to the surgeon general's report, the lower Medicaid participation rates have been linked to mistaken beliefs among immigrants that enrolling in Medicaid jeopardizes applications for citizenship.

With statistics indicating that America's mental health crisis is widespread and growing, and disparities in the Asian American community beginning to be recognized, in 1999, NAWHO began to focus on a population that was particularly at risk—college-age Asian American women. I'm so grateful for the contributions of the NAWHO Mental Health Advisory Committee, NAWHO Board Chair Dr. David Takeuchi and Dr. Henry Chung who were instrumental in the early stages of this survey. Their help was invaluable.

The NAWHO study, called *Breaking the Silence*, conducted a series of eleven focus groups from October of 1999 through May of 2000 with undergraduate Asian American women students between the ages of eighteen and thirty-four who were currently enrolled at San Francisco Bay Area colleges and universities. The study revealed that college-age Asian American women are at high risk for depression due to low levels of perceived life control and self-esteem, conditions that are closely linked to depression.

"High suicide rates don't surprise me because you feel so torn between your life and your parents' lives," said one twenty-year-old Asian American student at Diablo Valley College.

This comment offers insight into the conflicting cultural values that impact Asian American women's sense of control over their life decisions. Most of the focus group participants said they were in conflict with their families over women's roles, academic pursuits, and lifestyle issues such as dating driven by differences in the Asian and American cultures.

"There's a structure my parents expect me to live by, but the reality is that it doesn't always fit with the American culture I am growing up in," said one twenty-year-old at the University of California at Berkeley (UC Berkeley).

The cultural standards of the parents promote an unquestioned authority of the older generation and life paths for each family member based on gender. Daughters are expected to marry and care for their family while sons are expected to have careers and carry on the family name. The double standard is further conflicting for females because the culture demands achievement in education from everyone—however, for a daughter academic success is simply viewed as a way to find the perfect husband.

This set of circumstances creates emotionally charged conflicts of values and aspirations. On the other side of the coin, *Breaking the Silence* speculates that Asian parents have their own set of mental health stresses in dealing with the generation and cultural gap that exists with their children.

Since immigrant Asian American parents typically have sacrificed so much to support their children, many focus group participants said they felt guilty and obliged to fulfill their parents' dreams over their own. So, instead of pursuing careers they are interested in, they succumb to their parents' wishes and pursue professional careers such as medicine that their parents view as "safe."

"It's a battle going on in my head," said one eighteen-year-old participant from UC Berkeley. "I want to make my parents happy, but I want to be happy, too."

Similar to my own experience when I came to America with my family, several of the study participants said they were also stressed because they had such great responsibility within the family.

"Asian American women have more responsibilities than males," a nineteen-year-old from the University of California at Davis said. "You don't have a childhood growing up. You're already a parent [to other family members]."

The myth of the model minority also heaps on more pressure. Participants said they felt isolated and inferior because of the assumption that they should be smart and that they should know everything. Participants said this stereotype made them feel isolated on campus because they were held to high, unattainable academic standards.

While crisis lines and other mental health services certainly exist on college campuses, participants felt that the stigma and silence surrounding health issues, particularly mental health, in the Asian American culture kept them from accessing services.

"Asian American women are not educated about stress. Because of our culture, we're told we have to cover everything, but we're not told how to cope with it," said a nineteen-year-old student at San Francisco City College.

And similar to the many other health problems affecting the Asian American community, participants said that health care providers were not culturally competent or sensitive to their specific needs.

As I learned more about the problems of depression and suicide in the Asian American community, my focus began to turn to American society in general and the connection between prevailing attitudes and the great disparity in spending on mental health. A recent national survey showed that 71 percent of Americans believe that mental health problems are caused by emotional weakness; 65 percent believe they result from bad parenting; and 43 percent feel they are brought on in some way by the individual.

These misguided attitudes perpetuate the shame and stigma associated with mental illness and, as a result, quell public support for effective remedies. Only 7 percent of health spending in the United States goes to mental health services, and more than two-thirds of adults with diagnosable mental health problems go without treatment.

Of course the first step toward reducing the shame and stigma associated with mental illness and suicide is understanding and talking about the risks.

What Are the Risk Factors for Suicide?

According to the National Institute of Mental Health, researchers believe that both depression and suicide can be linked to decreased serotonin in the brain because low levels of serotonin have been detected in people who have attempted suicide as well as in suicide victims. Serotonin receptors in the brain increase their activity in persons with major depression and suicidal behavior. Currently studies are underway to evaluate medications that desensitize these receptors.

Other research suggests that familial and genetic factors contribute to the risk for suicidal behavior. Major psychiatric disorders such as bipolar disorder, major depression, schizophrenia, alcoholism and substance abuse, and some personality disorders are believed to run in families.

Of course that doesn't mean that you will commit suicide if someone in your family has, but it probably means that you are more vulnerable and should get evaluation and treatment if you exhibit any signs of mental illness.

What Are the Signs of Mental Illness?

Some of the common signs of mental illness may include:

- ◆ Prolonged or severe depression
- ◆ Marked personality change
- ◆ Flat or inappropriate emotions
- ◆ Undue, continuing anxiety and worry

- Tension-caused physical problems
- Withdrawal from society, isolation
- Hallucinations or delusions
- Unjustified fears
- Thoughts of suicide
- Rage or violence
- Obsessions or compulsions
- Substantial, rapid weight gain or loss
- Too much or too little sleep
- Excessive self-centeredness
- Loss of touch with reality
- Extremely immature behavior
- Negative self-image and outlook
- Inability to cope, overcome problems, stay in school, hold a job, or take care of one's own personal needs.[10]

Encouraging a better understanding of mental illness and suicide can help reduce the stigma that discourages individuals and their families from getting the help they need. Every day, each of us can help to reduce the stigma that surrounds mental illness by being aware of and altering our own behavior.

Do use respectful language to talk about people with psychiatric disorders.

Do emphasize abilities, not limitations.

Do tell someone if they are expressing a stigmatizing attitude.

Don't portray successful persons with disabilities as super human.

Don't use generic labels such as "retarded," or "the mentally ill."

Don't use terms like "crazy," "lunatic," "manic," "psycho" or "slow" to describe people with psychiatric disorders.[11]

By working to educate the public, I believe we can change the focus from the staggering statistics to the great hope for prevention and recovery that exists in the mental health field today. As NAWHO got more deeply involved in this important mental health work, my own interests began to widen beyond the Asian American community. It seemed that once again a cause—this time mental health and suicide prevention—was finding me.

After helping raise more than $14 million for NAWHO and establishing it as a leading health organization with more than eleven successful projects, it was time for me to take on new challenges. While at NAWHO, I had worked to elevate the status of Asian American women's health. I had served as the CEO for eight years, and it was truly a wonderful experience. In December of 2000, I stepped down as the CEO of NAWHO and went on to work for the American Public Health Association and other prominent health care projects.

US Surgeon General David Satcher, M.D., Ph.D. appointed me to serve on the Steering Committee of the Campaign to Eliminate Racial and Ethnic Disparities in Health, a partnership between the US Department of Health and Human Services and the American Public Health Association. This work evolved into a consulting position for the surgeon general's National Strategy for Suicide Prevention. I was blessed with the leadership opportunities at these organizations, and this fulfilling work helped my interest in mental heath intensify.

In June of 2001, I decided to start another project, with a focus on mental health and youth suicide prevention. Although I still serve as a consultant to several other health organizations, the new organization I founded, the Iris Alliance Fund, is the project I now use to promote suicide prevention. I guess I just don't want to let go of my older sister. I created the fund in my sister's memory taking as a symbol one of her favorite flowers, a flower that represents life, hope, and new beginnings.

CHAPTER TWELVE

Celebration

The Work Continues

Anniversaries are a time to take stock, to measure progress, and to set new goals. As I write this book, NAWHO prepares to celebrate its tenth anniversary as a strong and growing national voice working to eliminate health disparities in the Asian American community. And my other labor of love, the Iris Alliance Fund, is also gaining momentum with its message of hope. I am so proud of the work of both of these organizations, and how they continue to enrich my life.

There are also personal reasons for celebration. In 2000, after ten years of attending college classes and studying at night and on weekends to receive my bachelor's degree from the University of San Francisco, I earned my MBA in Golden Gate University's Executive MBA program. Though I had successfully built a large, national organization, I had always felt that I needed more business skills. The program helped me to formalize my thinking, giving me new approaches to organizational development and business planning.

I am so thankful to have many things to celebrate in my life, and one of those celebrations came on September 10,

2001, when *Redbook* magazine honored me as one of its "Mothers and Shakers" for "shattering the myth of the model minority." I had been recognized along with NAWHO by other publications, but this was the first mainstream national publication to acknowledge the difference NAWHO was making for Asian American women. Senator Hillary Rodham Clinton, who was also being honored "for shaking up the entire health care establishment," was the keynote speaker at a luncheon at Lincoln Center.

I was so emotional when I walked into Lincoln Center that day and was thankful to have my fiancé, Dennis Hayashi, with me to share the experience.

In October, Dennis and I were going to be married. I had met him when I first moved to San Francisco, and he had long been one of my role models. He was an attorney with the Asian American civil rights organization that I worked for as a bookkeeper. I always admired him because he had dedicated his life to helping other people and working against social injustice. When I was only beginning to learn about needs in the Asian American community, Dennis was successfully representing Asian Americans who had suffered great injustice.

Dennis has such a quiet strength that is completely endearing. We had been engaged since December of 1999 when he let me know in his unassuming way that he was thinking about asking me to marry him. Dennis and I had dated for years, and, each year at Christmastime, he always asked me what I wanted from him. But in 1999, as we shopped together for friends and family, I realized that he had not yet asked.

"Dennis, you haven't asked me what I want for Christmas yet," I reminded him, in my typically direct way.

"Well," he said, "I was thinking of getting you a ring."

"What kind of ring?" I asked.

"A little diamond," he answered.

Not realizing exactly where this was going, I asked him what kind of little diamond, and when Dennis answered simply, "a solitaire," I said somewhat incredulously, "like an engagement ring?"

Still not stating the obvious, he simply said, "Yes, like an engagement ring."

It was a wonderful Christmas present. But far more important than the ring, I was becoming a part of Dennis's family, who I already dearly loved. Part of the reason that Dennis has given his whole life to civil rights work is that his parents were both interned during World War II. Dennis's father, George Hayashi, was born in Seattle. His parents operated a mom and pop grocery store. During the Depression, they moved to Bainbridge Island in the Puget Sound and worked as farmers with fifty other Japanese families. When World War II started, George was a sophomore studying engineering at the University of Washington.

When Pearl Harbor was bombed on December 7, 1941, the lives of the Hayashi family, along with Japanese families across the country, were changed. Bainbridge Island was close to a highly sensitive communications station as well as a naval yard. The Hayashi's were one of the first families to be evacuated and interned at Manzanar, a hastily erected tar-papered military barrackstown for ten thousand below the east slope of Mount Whitney.

Since he was born a US citizen and was of legal draft age, George had a draft classification. His was 1-C, which was a limited service classification because of an inquinal hernia. After his internment, he was reclassified to the alien classification of 4-C. After a year of incarceration, the government eased restrictions and George was permitted to go to Colorado where he met his future wife, Yuki, who had also been interned with her family in Utah.

On V-E day, May 5, 1945, George was in the hospital recovering from having his hernia repaired. Shortly thereafter, he got a notice from the draft board—he was 1-A and would soon be sent to the Army Air Corp. He was honorably discharged in September of 1947 as a buck sergeant.

After he and Yuki were married in 1948 they raised three children, my husband Dennis, and his younger brother and sister, Gary and Dee. He was an engineer at the Department of Water and Power for forty-one years and a faithful and active member of his church. George's experiences certainly shaped those of his family, but also those around him. When he died at the age of eighty, four months after Dennis and I were married, hundreds attended his funeral.

I was so glad that George was able to celebrate his first son's wedding. Dennis married me late in his life, and so everyone in his family had given up on him! Dennis's father made a home video of the three siblings, Dennis, Gary, and Dee, when they were little children. The footage of them at Disneyland and on other family vacations shows these wonderful and caring parents in action. Dennis is so much like his father—responsible, hard working, caring, and passionate about helping others. Knowing that Dennis grew up in a small, three-bedroom apartment in Los Angeles, and knowing the discrimination and resulting financial hardships his parents overcame, I can see that he was destined to give nearly thirty years to public service.

These are just a few of the reasons why I felt so humble being honored by *Redbook* in 2001 with Dennis by my side.

Also the occasion gave Dennis an opportunity to meet one of his boyhood idols—a complete surprise.

There were many other amazing women being recognized that day at the luncheon. Heather Mills, who was being distinguished for her work with land mine victims, was going to present my award. But I didn't know that Dennis and I would be sitting with her and her soon-to-be husband. When we found our table, Paul McCartney was already seated there. Dennis, who is a big Beatles fan, couldn't believe it. Dennis is a great music lover and has an extensive music collection with everything ever recorded by the Beatles. Being able to sit with Paul McCartney was icing on the cake that day. When I sat down, he asked me how I was doing, and I said, "I'm very nervous, I think because you're sitting right here and talking to me."

So, he said, "Well, then let me sing to you."

He sang a verse of "I want to hold your hand" while holding my hand to calm my nerves. Which of course made me speechless.

When the time came for me to take the stage with Heather Mills, my focus was not on the incredible women who were at the luncheon, or on Paul McCartney, but on someone who was not there—my sister Bo Yoon.

My sister's voice fell silent in 1980, but on September 10, 2001, I spoke for her. I felt privileged not only to be able to change my life, control my own destiny and pursue my own dreams but also to be in a position to help other people who needed someone to speak for them until they could find their own voice. On that day especially, I knew that my sister's death meant something. Even though the pictures of her were gone, even though all of her belongings had been burned, she was still very much alive with me.

Of course the next morning, the whole world changed when terrorists attacked New York and Washington, DC. Dennis and I were waiting for a car to go to the airport when we heard the news about the tragedy at the World Trade Center. We ended up staying in New York for a week, in shock along with the rest of the city, watching the images on television in disbelief on September 11. The streets were filled with people—there were no cars, no taxi cabs. The normally deafening clamor of honking and shouting was silenced—no one was even talking. And everyone was heading in one direction—off the island of Manhattan. It was surreal. The emotions of that day were raw and numbing. I had been in a meeting with a friend at 120 Wall Street the night before, and I kept thinking how I had just been there and now it was gone. Months later Paul McCartney wrote about his 9/11 experiences for a major magazine. It's hard to believe that so much time has passed since 9/11, and I hope that those who lost loved ones that day have found peace.

I know a little bit about finding peace in the wake of grief. And, through the work of the Iris Alliance Fund, I plan to learn more. The essence of the work of the Iris Alliance Fund is hope. By increasing knowledge and awareness of depression and suicide through public education and working to reduce the silence and stigma, we can save lives.

Starting the Iris Alliance Fund was much different from starting NAWHO. Endorsements and support came more easily this time. People knew my work with NAWHO, and I was truly honored that some of the people on the NAWHO Board of Directors decided to join the new effort. California First Lady Sharon Davis helped to launch the project, and David Satcher became our honorary chairman of the board in October of 2002. My dear colleague Mary Woolley from

Research!America had just lost her nephew to suicide when I went to talk to her about her serving on the Iris Alliance Fund Board of Directors. Many prominent leaders from Washington, DC—Debra Ness, Kathy Bonk, Phyllis Greenberger, and Lauren LeRoy—joined the organization all without hesitation. Many supporters accepted my invitation to join the work to improve mental health: Dr. Iris Litt, Steve Peeps, Dr. Henry Foster, Kathy Hamilton, Cynthia Gomez, and many other leaders. The NAWHO Board of Directors also provided seed money to start the Iris Alliance Fund. I especially thank David Takeuchi, Yishin Kuo, Pam Anderson, and Michelle Akina for having confidence in me. I will always be so grateful for that. The first outside startup funding came from Brenda Drake at the Goldman Fund, a friend who supported me when I was at NAWHO for eight years. Deidre Lind, my good friend at Kaiser Permanente, also supported the Iris Alliance Fund early on in its development.

The work of the Iris Alliance Fund is just beginning with a focus on educating the public and stakeholders about mental health issues, breaking down misperceptions, and eliminating stigma and discrimination. We also are beginning to develop partnerships with community leaders to promote innovation and best practices in prevention, and to strengthen community and family environments that enhance protective factors for children. To accomplish these goals, we've started to raise money and have organized a national advisory board of sixty prominent leaders. I'm proud that in 2003, Tipper Gore spoke at the Iris Alliance Fund's second annual meeting.

Over the last decade, I have learned many lessons. To truly break the stigma surrounding mental illness, again the work comes back to "breaking the silence." To build a healthier country, we must share knowledge, talk about taboos, train health care providers, and let go of the culture of silent suffering that works against health and well being. We must do this in our everyday lives. Even those who are educated, empowered, and part of the movement sometimes have trouble letting go of the old ways. They shy away from confrontation and are still being controlled by tradition.

I certainly don't have all of the answers—none of us does. And so the work continues. To truly be agents of change, we must all take responsibility for our own health and our own lives. In the Asian American community, partnership and intervention activities are still needed to reduce the great disparities that put this population at risk. But these initiatives will only become a powerful force for positive change as long as Asian Americans refuse complacency.

I've always known that I didn't have to play with the cards I was dealt, and, as a result, much of my life's work has been letting other people know that's true for them as well.

When I was five years old, my father sometimes was a guest host of a live television talk show. One week there was a singing contest, and I wanted to be a part of it. I memorized my songs, and my father let me be on the show. There I stood before the audience and cameras, this tiny girl wearing a velvet dress and little black shoes. As the band played the introduction, I started singing too early. So I turned to these men and told them to stop and to start over. They were astonished, as were the audience and my father, at this little girl telling adult men what to do. I stood my ground even though everyone in the audience was laughing. I waited, fully expecting them to do as I said. When they did, I sang my song.

This was not the Korean way. But I hadn't learned the traditions yet. I just wanted to sing.

I think we all have that little girl inside of us—the person deep within that thinks for herself or himself and says what he or she thinks. I know that I am resisting what tradition and culture and society are trying to make me become.

The message of hope is that we can all be like that little girl. If we don't like our lives, we don't have to give up. We can change. We can grow.

Notes

Chapter 1

1   Robert Nilson, *Moon Handbooks: South Korea*, second edition (Avalon Travel Publishing, Inc., 1997) 638–40.

2   Rachel Simmons, *Odd Girl Out: The Hidden Culture of Aggression in Girls* (Harcourt, 2002) 3.

Chapter 4

1   P. Ong, *The State of Asian American America: Economic Diversity, Issues, and Policies (Los Angeles: LEAP, 1994).*

2   *Profile of Women's Health Status in California 1984–1994* (CA DHS Office of Women's Health, 1997).

3   E. Richard Brown et al., *Women's Health-Related Behaviors and Use of Clinical Preventive Services: A Report to The Commonwealth Fund* (Los Angeles: UCLA Center for Health Policy Research, 1995).

4   Centers for Disease Control and Prevention, National Center for Health Statistics, *Health, United States 1995* (Hyattsville, MD: US Public Health Service, 1994).

5   Center for the American Woman and Politics, *National Information Bank on Women in Public Office* (Eagleton Institute of Politics, Rutgers University); *Women of Color in Elective Office* (New Brunswick, NJ: Center for the American Woman and Politics, 1997).

Chapter 5

1   United States Congress, Office of Technology Assessmen, *Hip Fracture Outcomes in People Age 50 and Over: Background Paper*, OTA-BP-H-120 (Washington, DC: Government Printing Office, 1994).

2   National Osteoporosis Foundation, National Osteoporosis Risk Assessment Press Release, "Study of Postmenopausal Women Showed Hispanics, Asians and Native Americans May be at Greater Risk," www.nof.org (December 1998).

3   National Institute of Diabetes and Digestive and Kidney - Diseases (NIDDK) "Lactose Intolerance," www.niddk.nih.gov/

health/ digest/pubs/lactose/lactose.htm (April 1994; updated November 1998).

4 Centers for Disease Control and Prevention, National Center for Health Statistics, *National Health Interview Survey*, 1997.

5 E. A. Chrischilles et al., "A Model of Lifetime Osteoporosis Impact," *Archives of Internal Medicine* 151/10 (October 1991) 2026–32.

6 N. Ray et al., "Medical Expenditures for the Treatment of Osteoporotic Fractures in the United States in 1995: Report from the National Osteoporosis Foundation," *Journal of Bone and Mineral Research* 12/1 (January 1997) 24–35.

7 V. Matkovic et al., "Timing of Peak Bone Mass in Caucasian Females and its Implication for the Prevention of Osteoporosis," *Journal of Clinical Investigation* 93 (1994) 799–808.

8 H. A. McKay et al., "Lifestyle Determinants of Bone Mineral: A Comparison Between Prepubertal Asian- and Caucasian-Canadian Boys and Girls," *Calcified Tissue International*, 16/5 (May 2000) 320–24.

9 L. K. Bachrach et al., "Decreased Bone Density in Adolescent Girls with Anorexia Nervosa," *Pediatrics* 86 (1990) 440–47.

Chapter 6

1 American Public Health Association, *Campaign to Eliminate Racial and Ethnic Disparities in Health, 2002,* 27.

2 The National Center for Health Statistics, Centers for Disease Control and Prevention, *Cigarette Smoking Among Adults— United States, 1994,* MMWR 45 (1996) 558–90.

3 US Bureau of Census, 1998.

4 The Nation Center for Health Statistics, Centers for Disease Control and Prevention, *Annual Smoking-Attributable Mortality, Years of Potential Life Lost, and Economic Costs—United States, 1995–1999,* MMWR 51 (2002) 14.

Chapter 7

1 B. A. Miller et al., eds., *Racial/Ethnic Patterns of Cancer in the United States 1988–1992,* NIH Pub. No. 96–41–4 (Bethesda, MD: National Cancer Institute, 1996).

2 American Cancer Society, California Division, and Public Health Institute, California Cancer Registry, *California Facts and*

Figures, 2001 (Oakland, CA: American Cancer Society, California Division, 2000).

3 L. A. G. Ries et al., eds., *Cancer Statistics Review, 1973–1996* (Bethesda, MD: National Cancer Institute, 1999).

4 "NAWHO Communicating Across Boundaries: A Cultural Competency Training on Breast and Cervical Cancers in Asian American Women," Training Curriculum, Unit I, Section 2, page 9.

5 K. Roe, as adapted from David Chen, San Jose State University, 1993.

6 C. Roat, "Bridging the Gap" Interpreter Training Program, Cross Cultural Health Care Program, www.diversityrx.org/html/moipr3.htm, 2000.

7 Cross Cultural Health Care Program, Code of Ethics, www.xculture.org/interpreter/overview/ethics.html, 2000.

Chapter 8

1 Office of Financial Management, State of Washington, 1999.

2 National Diabetes Education Program, *Diabetes and Asian Americans and Pacific Islanders Fact Sheet* (Bethesda, MD: National Institutes of Health, 1999).

3 Centers for Disease Control and Prevention, *National Diabetes Fact Sheet: National Estimates and General Information on Diabetes in the United States*, revised edition (Atlanta: US Department of Health and Human Services, Centers for Disease Control and Prevention, 1998).

4 National Center for Health Statistics, Centers for Disease Control and Prevention, *1986–1990 National Health Interview Survey* (Hyattsville, MD: US Public Health Service, 1996).

5 W. Y. Fujimoto et al., "Prevalence of Diabetes Mellitus and Impaired Glucose Tolerance Among Second-Generation Japanese American Men," *Diabetes* 36 (1987) 721–29.

6 E. S. K. Choi et al., "The Prevalence of Cardiovascular Risk Factors Among Elderly Chinese Americans," *Archives of Internal Medicine* 150 (1990) 413–18.

7 Hawaii Diabetes Control Program. Based on M. Wen, "Unpublished Analysis of Data from the Behavioral Risk Factor Surveillance System (BRFSS) from 1988–1995" (Atlanta: US Department of Health and Human Services, Centers for Disease Control and Prevention, 1998).

8   American Diabetes Association, *Women and Diabetes* (Alexandria, VA: American Diabetes Association, 2001).

9   American Diabetic Association, "Diabetes in Children," www.diabetes.org, 2001.

10   Centers for Disease Control and Prevention, *Chronic Disease in Minority Populations* (Atlanta: Centers for Disease Control and Prevention, 1992).

11   The Commonwealth Fund 2001 Health Care Quality Survey.

12   NAWHO Fall Edition, 1999.

13   A. Hosler, "A Recognition of Need—The Burden of Diabetes in Asian American Communities," NAWHO New York Diabetes Symposium, 2001.

14   American Heart Association, "Asian/Pacific Islanders and Cardiovascular Diseases: Biostatistical Fact Sheet," 1999.

Chapter 9

1   F. L. Sonnenstein et al., *Involving Males in Preventing Teen Pregnancy* (California: The Urban Institute, 1997).

2   S. Loue, L. S. Lloyd, and E. Phoombour, *Organizing Asian Pacific Islanders in an Urban Community to Reduce HIV Risk: A Case Study*, AIDS Education and Prevention 8 (5), 381–93, 1996.

3   Centers for Disease Control and Prevention, *Sexually Transmitted Disease Surveillance*, 1998.

4   B. A. Miller et al., eds., *Racial/Ethnic Patterns of Cancer in the United States 1998–1992*, NIH Pub. No. 96–4104 (Bethesda, MD: National Cancer Institute, 1996).

5   F. Xavier Bosch, "Prevalence of Human Papillomavirus in Cervical Cancer: A Worldwide Perspective," *Journal National Cancer Institute* 87/11 (1995).

6   *Cancer Facts and Figures 2002*, American Cancer Society, 2002.

Chapter 10

1   Letter from the Office of the Attorney General, www.ojp.usdoj.gov/vawo.

2   American Medical Association, "Facts About Sexual Assault" (1995–2000), www.ama-assn.org/public/releases/assault/facts.htm.

3   P. Tjaden and N. Thoennes, *Prevalence, Incidence, and Consequences of Violence against Women: Findings from the National Violence against Women Survey* (Atlanta: National Institute of Justice, Centers for Disease Control and Prevention, 1999) 1–16.

4   B. S. Fisher et al., "Crime in the Ivory Tower: The Level and Sources of Student Victimization," *Criminology* 36 (1998) 671–99.

5   "Violence by Intimates: Analysis of Data on Crime by Current or Former Spouses, Boyfriends, and Girlfriends." *Bureau of Justice Statistics Fact Book* (Washington, DC: U. S. Department of Justice, Office of Justice Programs, 1998) 13.

6   Asian Task Force Against Domestic Violence, "About the Asian Task Force" (2000), www.atask.org/about_atask.html.

7   A. Moon and O. Williams, "Perceptions of Elder Abuse and Help-Seeking Patterns among African American, Caucasian American, and Korean American Elderly Women," *Gerontologist* 33 (1993) 386–95.

8   Francis Cullen, Bonnie Fisher, and Michael Turner, *The Sexual Victimization of College Women* (US Department of Justice Office of Justice Programs, Bureau of Justice Statistics Special Report, December 2000) 29.

9   P. Tjaden and N. Thoennes, op. cit., 1–16.

Chapter 11

1   www.surgeongeneral.gov/library/mentalhealth/home.html.

2   Ibid.

3   www.mentalhealthcommission.gov/reports/FinalReport/FullReport.htm.

4   W. Kuo, "Prevalence of Depression among Asian Americans," *Journal of Nervous and Mental Disease* 172 (1984) 449–57.

5   D. W. Sue and A. Frank, "A Typical Approach to the Psychosocial Study of Chinese and Japanese American College Males," *Journal of Social Issues* 20 (1973) 142–48.

6   L. Harris & Associates, Inc., *The Commonwealth Fund Survey of the Health of Adolescent Girls*, 1997.

7   www.surgeongeneral.gov/library/mentalhealth/cre/fact2.asp.

8   Ibid.

9   www.surgeongeneral.gov/library/mentalhealth/cre/release.asp.

10   www.wyami.org/signs.htm.

11   Substance Abuse and Mental Health Services Administration National Mental Health Information Center, www. mentalhealth.org/cmhs.

Acknowledgments

When I began this project four years ago, I had several goals in mind. First, I wanted to draw attention to the significant gaps in the knowledge of health information about Asian American women. I also wanted to increase the utilization of NAWHO research and educational materials by policymakers, community leaders, health care professionals, and women's health organizations. And, most importantly, I wanted to make this information available to a broader audience.

At the time, there was no other book like this on the market. I was working without a net. Initially, my focus was only on the important statistics NAWHO had amassed as well as on the lessons we learned as we grew. But, as I began the process of gathering materials and writing, I learned that my reasons for starting NAWHO and my personal story were also important to share with the readers. Almost everyone I met through NAWHO had asked me not only how but also why I started the organization.

The process of writing this book actually was much like starting a new organization. I needed so much support along the way—someone to help research information, to edit, publish, finance, and endorse. I also needed many others to provide constant support and encouragement. And I definitely needed someone to talk to daily about the project, to share ideas as the book evolved.

Throughout the process, my hope was always that this book would inspire other Asian American women to share their stories so that we can all learn more about our health and well being. I knew that if we could pull back the cloak of silence that surrounds the Asian American community, more

Asian American women would emerge as advocates for important social change.

It has taken four years to finally publish *Far From Home*, and I have many people to thank for making the book possible. First, my publisher, Jill Bertolet, and Sally Giddens Stephenson. Your guidance and insight were invaluable, and I could not have finished this book without the two of you.

I want to thank Afton Kobayashi, who was the second staff member at NAWHO and who was with me every step of the way for nine years as we raised funds and created programs. I will be forever appreciative of her unwavering commitment to NAWHO, first as program coordinator, then as communications director and finally as executive director.

NAWHO has been enriched by the efforts of many volunteers and NAWHO National Leadership Network members who have given their time and support over the past ten years to work for positive change.

I want to acknowledge the essential efforts of the 2003 NAWHO Board of Directors; Dr. David Takeuchi, chair; Robin Chin, former chair; Sarah Lee; Tina Lee; Dr. YiShin Kuo; Dr. Pam Anderson; Dr. Marion Lee; Rebecca Sze; Dr. Descarti Li; and Dr. Henry Chung. And all of the NAWHO staff members with special thanks to the leadership team: Karen Lim, communications director; Jennifer Stoll Hayadia, former director of programs; Michelle Akina, director of finance and administration; and, of course, Afton.

Also Priya Jagannathan, who came to work for me at NAWHO when I had nothing. She volunteered for more than eight months while she was a student at the University of California Berkeley studying for her master's degree in public health. When NAWHO finally had the funding, she became a staff member and served as our first program director for four years. Bill Wong has also been a significant NAWHO supporter. He volunteered for NAWHO for many years, generously donating his time for our graphic design needs. Bill also gave us our first computer and, even though he was extremely busy with his work in the California legislature, he was always available to help sell tickets for our fundraisers or to provide invaluable moral support to everyone at NAWHO.

Also many thanks to everyone who contributed to creating NAWHO publications and program materials, which provided valuable information used throughout this book.

I'm grateful to Robert Ausura, who was the creative mind behind the title *Far From Home.* Over the years Robert has been a trusted advisor on various writing projects.

I want to recognize the many people and organizations who believed in the vision of NAWHO:

Startup funders Shira Saperstein and The Moriah Fund; Jael Silliman and the Jessie Smith Noyes Foundation; The Sister Fund; Michele Lord and the Norman Foundation; and The Church Women United.

Major funders of NAWHO's projects: Brenda Drake and the Richard and Rhoda Goldman Fund; the Ford Foundation; the Kellogg Foundation; the Hewlett Foundation; Adisa Douglas and the Public Welfare Foundation; Deidre Lind and Kaiser Permanente.

Over the past decade, the Centers for Disease Control and Prevention (CDC) has played a leading role in NAWHO's efforts as a partner on many groundbreaking health initiatives. Many of our cooperative efforts were the first initiatives of their kind to focus on Asian American women. These cooperative agreements have included the National Center for Chronic Disease Prevention Division of Cancer Prevention and Control, Division of Diabetes Translation, Office on Smoking and Health, and National Immunization Program as well as the National Center for Injury Prevention and Control Division of Violence Prevention.

We have also been fortunate to have cooperative agreements with the Substance Abuse and Mental Health Services Administration Center for Substance Abuse Prevention and the National Institutes of Health Osteoporosis and Related Bone Diseases National Resource Center.

I want to thank all of the CDC projects officers for their day-to-day guidance as we implemented these important programs. And I want to express my gratitude to Dr. Jim Marks, director of the National Centers for Chronic Disease Prevention, and Dr. David Satcher, former director of the CDC and former surgeon general of United States. These two men have provided exceptional leadership in the work to eliminate health disparities in ethnic minority populations.

I also want to acknowledge the valuable leadership and support provided by US Representatives Nancy Pelosi, Patsy Mink, Robert Matsui and Anna Eshoo. I also appreciate the support of Tipper Gore, who honored NAWHO and me at the vice president's residence in April of 1999. When she asked me to invite one hundred people to the reception, I asked a hundred of the NAWHO National Leadership Network members to join us so that I could share the event with these emerging Asian American health advocates.

As I enter a new phase of advocacy work, I want to recognize the members of the Board of Directors of Iris Alliance Fund for their continuing help, especially, Robin Chin, Mary Woolley, Dian Harrison, and startup funder Brenda Drake and The Goldman Fund. For helping us launch the Iris Alliance Fund and for continuing to support our cause, I thank California First Lady Sharon Davis. She is a role model for women in California who has been working on mental health issues for many years. We are thankful that she has allowed us to name an important new award after her—the Iris Alliance Fund's Sharon Davis Award for Excellence in Leadership.

Along the way, I have been fortunate to have many colleagues and friends who were generous with their advice and support: Leticia Alejandrez, Marie Bass, Robin Chin, Brenda Drake, Gloria Feldt, Laura Flinchbaugh, Kitty Hsu Dana, Kathleen Hamilton, Kathy Kneer, Deidre Lind, Kate Michelman, Carol Jane, Sia Nowrojee, Julia Scott, Lilly Spitz, Terri Thomas, and Dian Harrison, whose can-do attitude has always inspired me to take action.

More recently, I had an opportunity to work with some exceptional leaders in Sacramento who are building the Capital Unity Center (CUC). Founded in 1999, CUC is an interactive learning and exhibition space commemorating California's diversity. The project got its start following hate crimes in the Sacramento area including three arsons at synagogues. I have learned so much from the leaders of this group, especially Assembly Member Darrell Steinberg, State Senator Deborah Ortiz, and all of the other CUC board members.

On a more personal note, for helping to shape my thoughts and actions, I am grateful to my parents. I especially appreciate my husband, Dennis Hayashi, who is a constant role model and inspiration. I've talked to him about the book almost every day for the past four years. He's the one who most encouraged me to write it.

Every day I am thankful for my sister and best friend Cindy Omiya and her son Nick Omiya. They both faithfully encourage me to face new challenges. And finally, I treasure my goddaughter, Tiffany Jade Chin, and my nephew, Nick—the children in my life and the best teachers I have.

Resources

NAWHO Publications
(In English)

*Expanding Options: A Reproductive and Sexual Health Survey of
Asian American Women*

*Making a Difference: Highlights from a National Symposia Series
on Asian Americans and Diabetes*

A Profile on Cervical Cancer and Asian American Women

*Global Perspectives: A Report on International Asian American
Women's Reproductive Health*

*Health Risks & Need For Prevention: A Tobacco Report on South-
east Asian Youth*

*Breaking The Silence: A Study of Depression among Asian Ameri-
can Women*

*Community Solutions: Meeting the Challenge of STDs in Asian
Americans and Pacific Islanders*

The Asian American Men's Health Study: Sharing Responsibility

*The Heart of the Community: A Profile on Asian American Women
and Heart Disease*

Smoking among Asian Americans: A National Tobacco Survey

*Learning from Communities: A Guide to Addressing the Reproduc-
tive Health Needs of Vietnamese American Women*

*National Plan of Action on Asian American Women and Breast
Cancer*

*Emerging Communities: A Health Needs Assessment of South
Asian Women in Three California Counties*

*Silent Epidemic: A Survey of Violence among Young Asian Ameri-
can Women*

Asian Language Health Education Materials

Breast and Cervical Cancer

Mammography (In Cambodian, Chinese, Thai, Vietnamese,
Korean, Laotian, or Tagalog)
Agency for Healthcare Research and Quality
2101 E. Jefferson Street, Suite 501
Rockville, MD 20852
Phone: (800) 358-9295
Web site: http://www.ahcpr.gov

Breast Cancer; Breast Self-Exam; Cervical Cancer (In Cambodian,
Chinese, Farsi, Japanese, Korean, Laotian, Tagalog, Tongan,
or Vietnamese)
American Cancer Society: California Division
1710 Webster St.
PO Box 2061
Oakland, CA 94604
Phone: (510) 452-5229

Breast Health (In Korean)
American Cancer Society: Eastern Division
Korean Outreach Program
NY, NY
Phone: (718) 263-1532
www.cancer.org

Breast Cancer; Breast Self-Exam; Breast Health; Mammography
(In Chinese)
American Cancer Society: Fremont, CA
Northern California Chinese Branch Unit
39277 Liberty Street, Suite D-14
Fremont, CA 94538
Phone: (510) 797-0600; (888) 566-6222

Breast Cancer (In Vietnamese)
American Cancer Society: Inland Empire area, CA
Desert Sierra Area
Phone: (909) 683-6415

Breast Cancer (In Tagalog)
American Cancer Society: Long Beach, CA
(562) 437-0797

Breast Cancer (In Chinese)
American Cancer Society: Los Angeles, CA
Phone: (310) 670-2650

Breast Health (In Cambodian, Hmong, Japanese, Korean, Laotian,
Tagalog, Thai, or Vietnamese)
American Cancer Society: Minnesota Division
3316 West 66th St.
Minneapolis, MN 55435
Phone: (800) ACS-2345
www.mn.cancer.org

Breast Self-Exam; Breast Cancer; Cervical Health; Cervical Cancer (In Chinese)
American Cancer Society: New York City, NY
Chinese American Cancer Association
41–25 Kissena Blvd, Room 103
Flushing, NY 11354
Phone: (718) 886-8890
Fax: (718) 886-8891
www.caca-acs.org

Breast Cancer (In Korean)
American Cancer Society: Orange County, CA
Alton Deere Plaza
1940 East Deere Ave. #100
Santa Ana, CA 92705
Phone: (949) 261-9446

Breast Cancer (In Chinese)
American Cancer Society: San Francisco, CA
San Francisco Chinatown Office
Phone: (415) 677-2458

Breast Cancer (In Vietnamese)
1715 S. Bascom Ave., Suite 100
Campbell, CA 95008
Phone: (408) 879-1032

Cancer Screening; Breast Health; Breast Self-Exam; Cervical Health; Pap Smear; Mammogram (In Bahasa (Malay), Cambodian, Chinese, Gujrati, Hmong, Indonesian, Japanese, Kannada, Korean, Laotian, Marathi, Persian (Farsi), Tagalog, Thai, or Vietnamese)
American Cancer Society: St. Paul, MN
3316 W. 66th Street
Minneapolis, MN 55435
Phone: (952) 925-2772
www.cancer.org

Breast Health; Cervical Health (In Korean)
Asian Health Services
Korean Women's Health Project
818 Webster Street
Oakland, CA 94607
Phone: (510) 986-6830
www.ahschc.org

Cervical Cancer (In Chinese or Vietnamese)
California Department of Health Services
Office of Women's Health
Sacramento, CA
www.dhs.ca.gov/director/owh

Breast Cancer; Mammogram (In Chinese, Tagalog, or
  Vietnamese)
  California Medical Review, Inc. (CMRI)
  One Sansome St., Suite 600
  San Francisco, CA 94104-4448
  Phone: (415) 677-2000
  Fax: (415) 677-2195
  www.cmri-ca.org

Breast Cancer Survivor video (In Hmong)
  Center for Hmong Arts and Talent and Frogtown
  Media Productions
  995 University Ave. West, #220
  St Paul, MN 55104
  Phone: (651) 603-6971

Breast Cancer; Breast Self-Exam; Pap Smear (In Chinese)
  Chinatown Health Clinic
  258 Canal Street, First Floor
  New York, NY 10013
  Phone: (212) 966-0228

Breast Cancer Resources and Support Groups (In Chinese)
  Chinatown Public Health Center
  San Francisco Dpt of Public Health
  1490 Mason St.
  San Francisco, CA 94133
  Phone: (415) 705-8500

Breast Cancer Diagnosis and Treatment (In Chinese)
  Chinese Community Cancer Information Center (In Chinese)
  835 Jackson St. Room 413
  San Francisco, CA 94133
  Phone: (415) 677-2458
  (415) 677-2457

Breast Self-Exam; Mammogram; Pap Smear (In Vietnamese)
Family Health Center of Worcester
26 Queen St.
Worcester, MA 01610
Phone: (508) 860-7700
www.fhcw.org

Breast Self-Exam (In Korean)
Korean Health Education, Information, and Referral Center
(KHEIR) Health Center
266 S. Harvard Blvd.
Los Angeles, CA 90006
Phone: (213) 637-1070
Fax: (323) 373-1080

Breast Self-Exam (In Korean)
Koryo Health Foundation
1058 South Vermont St.
Los Angeles, CA 90006
Phone: (213) 380-8833
Fax: (213) 368-6047

Breast Self-Exam video (In Chinese, Japanese, Korean, Tagalog,
or Vietnamese)
Lange Productions
7661 Curson Terrace
Hollywood, CA 90046
Phone: (888) LANGE-88

Breast Health; Pap Smear; Mammography (In Vietnamese)
National Cancer Institute-National Institutes of Health
PO Box 24128
Baltimore, MD 21227
Phone: (800) 422-6237
www.nci.nih.gov

Interpretations Available for Breast Cancer; Breast Self-Exam;
   Breast Cancer Treatment; Cervical Cancer (In Cambodian,
   Chinese, Japanese, Korean, Laotian, Thai, Vietnamese)
   Pacific Asian Language Services (PALS) for Health
   605 West Olympic Boulevard, Suite 600
   Los Angeles, CA 90015
   Phone: (213) 553-1818

Breast Health (In Vietnamese)
   Santa Clara Valley Breast Cancer Early Detection
      Partnership
   Phone: (408) 289-9974 or (800) 505-1818

Breast Cancer; Cervical Cancer (In Cambodian or Vietnamese)
   South Cove Community Health Center
   885 Washington Street
   Boston, MA 02111
   Phone: (617) 482-7555

Breast Exam; Mammogram; Pap Smear (In Chinese, Cambodian,
   Japanese, Korean, Tagalog, or Vietnamese)
   Union of Pan Asian Communities
   1031 Twenty-fifth Street
   San Diego, CA 92102
   Phone: (619) 531-8871 or (619) 235-4277
   Fax: (619) 235-9002

Pap Smear; Mammogram (In Cambodian Chinese, Korean, Lao-
   tian, Thai, or Vietnamese)
   US Department of Health and Human Services
   US Food and Drug Administration, Office of Women's
      Health
   600 Fishers Lane
   Rockville, MD 20857
   Some languages available on-line at www.apanet.org/~fdala

Breast Cancer; Pap Smear (In Cambodian, Chinese, Hmong,
    Korean, Laotian, Tagalog, Thai, or Vietnamese)
    Utah Department of Health
    Spencer S. Eccles Health Sciences Library
    University of Utah
    Health Science Center
    10 N. 1900 E.
    Salt Lake City, UT 84112-5890
    Phone: (801) 581-8771   Fax: (801) 581-3632
    medstat.med.utah.edu/library/refdesk/24lang.html

Breast Self-Exam; Cervical Health; Breast Health; Breast Cancer;
    Breast Cancer Treatment (In Vietnamese)
    Vietnamese Community Health Promotion Project—Univer-
        sity of California, San Francisco
    44 Montgomery Street, Suite 850
    San Francisco, CA 94104
    Phone: (415) 476-0557   Fax: (415) 956-6247
    Materials also available at: www.healthisgold.org
    Web site: medicine.ucsf.edu/divisions/vchpp

Breast Self-Exam (In Cambodian, Laotian, or Vietnamese)
    Vietnamese Mutual Assistance Association
    Asian Health Care Services
    1320 North Peak Street
    Dallas, TX 75204
    Phone: (214) 691-1704   Fax: (214) 696-0275
    http://hometown.aol.com/vmaatx/vmaa.html

Health Checklist For Women 50+ (includes mammogram and pap
    smear) (In Chinese)
    50+ and Strong
    Phone: (916) 658-0159
    www.50strong.org

*The American Cancer Society consolidated database of Asian
language materials is accessible through (800) ACS-2345.

Birth Control

Birth Control (In Chinese)
    Chinatown Health Clinic
    125 Walker Street, 2nd Floor
    New York, NY 10013
    Phone: (212) 226-1872

Birth Control (In Chinese)
    Chinatown Service Center, Family Planning Clinic
    600 N. Broadway
    Los Angeles, CA 90012
    Phone: (213) 972-8840

Birth Control (In Chinese, Korean, English-Cambodian, or
    English-Laotian)
    492 Division Street
    Campbell, CA 95008
    Phone: (408) 374-3720

Birth Control (In Cambodian, Laotian, or Vietnamese)
    Indochinese Cultural and Service Center/Indochinese Lan-
        guage Resource Center
    3030 Southwest Second Avenue
    Portland, OR 97201
    Phone: (503) 239-0132

Emergency Contraception (In Cambodian, Chinese, Korean, Lao-
    tian, or Vietnamese)
    Northwest Emergency Contraception Coalition
    PATH (Program for Appropriate Technology in Health)
    4 Nickerson Street
    Seattle, WA 98109
    Phone: (206) 285-3500 or (888) 668-2528
    Email: info@path.org
    www.path.org

Birth Control (In Korean or Laotian)
 T.H.E. Clinic, Asian Health Project
 3860 W. Martin Luther King Boulevard
 Los Angeles, CA 90008
 Phone: (323) 295-6571

Diabetes

Diabetes Care Card—"Know Your Blood Sugar Numbers" (In
 Chinese or Vietnamese)
 Massachusetts Health Promotion Clearinghouse
 (For Massachusetts residents)
 The Medical Foundation
 95 Berkeley Street
 Boston, MA 02116
 Phone: (800) 952-6637
 Fax: (617) 536-8012
 www.maclearinghouse.com

"You can do it"; "You Can Manage It" (In Cambodian, Chinese,
 Hmong, Korean, Laotian, Tagalog, or Vietnamese)
 National Diabetes Education Program
 http://ndep.nih.gov/conduct/psa-aapi.htm

"Food Guide: Diabetes before and after Pregnancy" (In Cambo-
 dian, Chinese, Hmong, Korean, Laotian, or Vietnamese)
 Sweet Success
 4542 Ruffner Street, Suite 130
 San Diego, CA 92111-2250
 Phone: (858) 467-4990
 Fax: (858) 467-4993

Health Checklist for Women 50+ (In Chinese)
 50+ and Strong
 Phone: (916) 658-0159
 www.50strong.org

Cancer

Taking Control (healthy habits) (In Korean)
American Cancer Society: Eastern Division (New York)
Korean Outreach Program
Phone: (718) 263-1532 or (800) ACS-2345
www.cancer.org

*The American Cancer Society consolidated database of Asian language materials is accessible through (800) ACS-2345.

Mental Health
For case managers that speak Asian languages:

Asian Counseling and Referral Services (ACRS)
720 8th Ave., South, Suite 200
Seattle, WA 98104-3006
Phone: (206) 695-7600
Fax: (206) 695-7606
Mental Health Intake Office: (206) 695-7511
www.acrs.org

Lao Family Community of Minnesota Health Center
320 W. University Ave.
St. Paul, MN 55103
Phone: (651) 221-0069
www.acmhs.org

Asian Health Services
818 Webster St.
Oakland, CA 94607
Phone: (510) 986-6830
www.ahschc.org

Support groups and workshops available (In Japanese or English)
Little Tokyo Service Center
231 E. 3rd Street, Suite G104
Los Angeles, CA 90013
Phone: (213) 473-1602
Fax: (213) 473-1601
Nikkei Helpline: (800) NIKKEI-1 or (213) 473-1633
www.ltsc.org

Reading references in Asian languages
Dementia (In Chinese)
Spencer S. Eccles Health Sciences Library
University of Utah Health Science Center
10 N. 1900 E.
Salt Lake City, UT 84112-5890
Phone: (801) 581-8771   Fax: (801) 581-3632
Materials are available through the following Web site:
http://medstat.med.utah.edu/library/refdesk/24lang.html

Drugs are all around us . . . Help your child avoid them (for parents) (In Cambodian, Chinese, Laotian, Tagalog, Vietnamese, or English)
Drugs are all around you . . . Can you live without them? (for youth) (In Cambodian, Chinese, Laotian, Tagalog, Vietnamese, or English)
Your Child's Mental Health (In Cambodian, Chinese, Korean, Japanese, Laotian, Tagalog, Vietnamese, or English)
Stress (in Chinese)
What is Depression? (In Chinese, Japanese, Vietnamese)
What is Schizophrenia? (In Chinese, Japanese, Vietnamese, English)
Available from:
Asian Community Mental Health Services
310 8th Street, Suite 201
Oakland, CA 94607
Phone: (510) 451-6729   Fax: (510) 268-0202

(In Chinese):
Attention-Deficit Hyperactivity Disorder in Children
Coping with the Loss of a Loved One—Grief & Bereavement
Depression: What you should know and what you can do about it
How to Live a Healthy Life—Fighting Depression
How to Promote Children's Emotional and Social Skills—For
    Parents
Learn to Cope with Stress and Trauma
Mental Health of Older Adults
Postpartum Depression
Stress
Teens: Coping with Stress

(In English):
Asian American Behavioral Health Service Directory for Metropoli-
    tan New York
Attention-Deficit Hyperactivity Disorder in Children
Coping with the Loss of a Loved One—Grief & Bereavement
Depression: What You Should Know and What You Can Do About It
How to Live a Healthy Life—Fighting Depression
How to Promote Children's Emotional and Social Skills—For
    Parents
Learn to Cope with Stress and Trauma
Postpartum Depression
Teens: Coping with Stress

Available from:
    Charles B. Wang Community Health Center
    125 Walker Street, 2nd Floor
    (212) 226-3888
    New York, NY, 10013
    Clinical Service: (212) 226-9339
    268 Canal Street
    New York, NY, 10013
    136–26 37th Ave., 2nd Floor
    Flushing, NY 11534

Understanding Depression (In Chinese or Vietnamese)
What is Post Traumatic Stress Disorder (PTSD)? (In Chinese or
   Vietnamese)

Available from:
   Asian Pacific Psychological Services
   431 30th Street, Suite 6A
   Oakland, CA 94609
   Phone: (510) 835-2777
   Fax: (510) 835-0164
   www.appsweb.org

Teens and Depression (In Korean)
Prevention of Depression (In Korean)
Prevention of Suicide (In Korean)
Post Traumatic Stress Disorder (PTSD) (In Vietnamese)

Available from:
   Center for Pan Asian Community Services, Inc
   3760 Park Avenue
   Doraville, GA 30340
   Phone: (770) 936-0969
   Fax: (770) 458-9377
   www.cpacs.org

*A Multilingual Mental Health Glossary and Resource Guide for
   Asian Americans* (In English, Cambodian, Chinese, Japanese, Korean, Laotian, Vietnamese)

Available from:
   Asian American Community Services (AACS)
   4100 North High St. Suite 301
   Columbus, OH 43214
   Phone: (614) 220-4023
   Interpreter's hotline: (614) 208-1298
   Fax: (614) 220-4024
   www.asiancomsv.org

About the Author

Iris Alliance Fund founder and president Mary Chung Hayashi has been called one of the "Mothers and Shakers of 2001" by *Redbook* Magazine, one of the "100 Most Influential Asian Americans of the Decade" by *A. Magazine*, a "Woman to Watch" by *Ladies' Home Journal*, and was a 2003 "Women and Industry" honoree by the Association of California Commissions for Women. She has advised the nation's top policy leaders, and has established unprecedented partnerships in support of social causes that previously had no financial or public backing.

Mary is the author of *Far From Home: Shattering the Myth of the Model Minority*. Part autobiography and part Asian American women's wellness guide, *Far From Home* is a groundbreaking book about the health of America's fastest growing community. Mary has also been a featured speaker at the California Governor's Women's Conference, The White House Conference on Mental Health, and the Annual Meeting of the Society for Public Health Education. She contributes her expertise to a number of other health policy initiatives, serving as a leadership consultant for the National Strategy for Suicide Prevention, as a steering committee member to the National Campaign to Eliminate Racial and Ethnic Disparities in Health, and as a SAMHSA Advisory Committee member. She has served as the campaign director to the American Public Health Association on their health disparities initiative, and is a trustee for Planned Parenthood Golden Gate, Research!America, the Institute for Diversity in Health Management, and the Alan Guttmacher Institute.

Mary has a Bachelor of Science degree in applied economics from the University of San Francisco, and a Master in Business Administration from Golden Gate University. She resides in Castro Valley, California with her husband, Dennis Hayashi, a noted civil rights attorney.

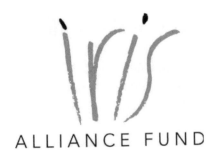

ALLIANCE FUND

About the Iris Alliance Fund

The Iris Alliance Fund is a mental health foundation that focuses on changing the public discourse to make youth suicide prevention a greater priority. The Iris Alliance Fund builds partnerships with public and private sector leaders to create new resources for mental health and provides funds to support effective community-based suicide prevention programs. Mary modeled the Iris Alliance Fund on the most successful elements of the National Asian Women's Health Organization (NAWHO), which she founded in 1993. Under her leadership, NAWHO grew into the nation's leading advocate for Asian American health issues, changing attitudes and polices regarding this underserved population through research, public education and community grant programs. Mary developed and directed over $10 million in national cooperative agreements with the Centers for Disease Control and Prevention, the Substance Abuse and Mental Health Services Administration, and the National Institutes of Health. Mary also fostered the leadership of more than three hundred young Asian American advocates by organizing an annual national leadership and public policy training program in Washington, DC, the first of its kind to focus on the health of Asian Americans.

Index